Occupational
Group Therapy

Occupational Group Therapy

Rosemary Crouch

School of Therapeutic Sciences, Faculty
of Health Sciences, University of
Witwatersrand, Johannesburg,
South Africa

WILEY Blackwell

Registered Office(s)
John Wiley & Sons, Inc., 111 River Street, Hoboken, NJ 07030, USA
John Wiley & Sons Ltd, The Atrium, Southern Gate, Chichester, West Sussex, PO19 8SQ, UK

Editorial Office
9600 Garsington Road, Oxford, OX4 2DQ, UK

For details of our global editorial offices, customer services, and more information about Wiley products visit us at www.wiley.com.

Wiley also publishes its books in a variety of electronic formats and by print-on-demand. Some content that appears in standard print versions of this book may not be available in other formats.

Library of Congress Cataloging-in-Publication Data

Names: Crouch, Rosemary B., author.
Title: Occupational group therapy / Rosemary B. Crouch.
Description: First edition. | Hoboken, NJ : Wiley-Blackwell, 2021. |
    Includes bibliographical references and index.
Identifiers: LCCN 2020044301 (print) | LCCN 2020044302 (ebook) | ISBN
    9781119591436 (paperback) | ISBN 9781119591443 (adobe pdf) | ISBN
    9781119591528 (epub)
Subjects: MESH: Occupational Therapy–methods | Psychotherapy,
    Group–methods
Classification: LCC RC487 (print) | LCC RC487 (ebook) | NLM WM 450.5.O2
    | DDC 616.89/165–dc23
LC record available at https://lccn.loc.gov/2020044301
LC ebook record available at https://lccn.loc.gov/2020044302

Cover Design: Wiley
Cover Image: © MirageC/Getty Images

Set in 10.5/13pt STIXTwoText by SPi Global, Pondicherry, India
Printed and bound by CPI Group (UK) Ltd, Croydon, CR0 4YY

C9781119591436_250321

This book is dedicated to my professional colleague
and great friend Vivyan Alers.

Vivyan was a respected and dedicated occupational therapist,
especially in group work, and much of her work is reflected
in this book.

She was involved initially as co-author of this book and was part of
the whole process of designing it and communicating with the
publishers. It was her dream to publish a book about her passion
for occupational group therapy. She was a skilled group therapist
and psychodramatist particularly in the use of the Therapeutic
Spiral technique. She used her skill in the most effective way when
she worked with impoverished and traumatised people in
Johannesburg as well as in many other environments.

She had an infectious and lovely, kind personality and was
much loved. She passed away suddenly at the age of 64 in 2018.
She is sadly missed.

— Rosemary Crouch

Contents

Author's Biographies

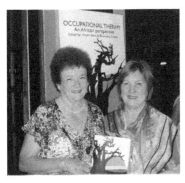

Rosemary Crouch and Vivyan Alers.

Rosemary Crouch

Dr. Rosemary Barncastle Crouch received her Diploma in Occupational Therapy from the University of Witwatersrand (Wits) in 1960 and graduated with a BSc. Occupational Therapy in 1971. She lectured in the Department of Occupational Therapy at Wits from 1973 until the end of 1989. She graduated with an MSc. with distinction at Wits in 1984. After leaving Wits at the end of 1989 she went into the private sector and was appointed as part-time senior lecturer in occupational therapy at MEDUNSA and Pretoria University. In 2003 she received her PhD at the Medical University of South Africa (MEDUNSA).

She has been appointed visiting lecturer to a number of universities including the University of Alberta in Edmonton in Canada in 2004. In 2007 she was appointed as a Mellon Mentor at Wits in the School of Therapeutic Sciences until the end of 2010. After a year of retirement she was appointed in 2012 to the Department of Nursing Education as a Mentor and appointed to the position of Honorary Adjunct Professor in the School of Therapeutic Sciences. She was also appointed in a part-time capacity to the Department of Research and School of Humanities at Wits until 2020.

Rosemary is the co-editor of three books with Vivyan Alers as co-author entitled 'Occupational Therapy in Psychiatry and Mental Health'. The fourth and fifth editions were published by Wiley & Blackwell Publishers (UK). She was also co-editor with Vivyan

Alers of the book 'Occupational Therapy: An African Perspective', published in Johannesburg by Shorten Publishers in 2010.

She edited a book entitled 'OTASA; A remarkable story' published by Sarah Shorten, in 2016. Rosemary has many publications in journals.

She held various positions in the Occupational Therapy Association of South Africa (OTASA) and was appointed OTASA Representative on the World Federation of Occupational Therapists (WFOT) for a total of 19 years. She was Chairman of the Education Committee of WFOT and then became Vice President for four years in 1998. In 2010 she was highly honoured to be awarded an Honorary Life Fellowship to WFOT.

She was chairperson of the Professional Board for Occupational therapy, Medical Orthotists and Prosthetists and Arts Therapists for eight years from 2004 to 2010. In 2019 she was honoured to be awarded a 'Health Merit Award' as a Top Professional by the Health Professions Council of South Africa (HPCSA).

She is an Honorary Life member of the Occupational Therapy Association of South Africa (OTASA).

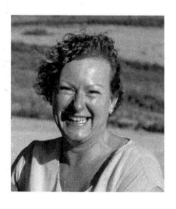

Louise Fouché
(Author of Chapter 4)

Louise qualified as an occupational therapist in 1992 at the University of Pretoria. She obtained a Post-graduate Diploma in Interpersonal Relationships and Group Activities with cum laude at the same university in 1999. In 2001 she received a Master's in Occupational Therapy in the Mental Health field (2001) at the University of Pretoria and a Post-graduate Certificate in Higher Education in 2004.

As a member of the Occupational Therapy Association of South Africa (OTASA), Louise was asked to lead the development of the scope of Group-work for the Occupational Therapy profession. This statement has been has been Gazetted.

Louise Fouché is the founder of 'OTGrow' a company that trains occupational therapists, both nationally and internationally, in specific group techniques which can be implemented with mental health care users. OTGrow was started 10 years ago and Louise has trained over 700 therapists to date. She was also instrumental in the development of St Raphael's Sanctuary's Healing Program that focuses on psycho-spiritual healing, which is unique as it merges psychological principals for healing with spiritual development, within a group context.

Louise has been instrumental in developing the Occupational Therapy Interactive Group Model (OTIGM) to a high level and many occupational group therapists have emerged as experts in this Model. It has been an important factor in the growth of occupational group therapy in South Africa and contributes greatly to the profession.

Preface

Footfalls echo in the memory,
down the passage we did not take,
towards the door we never opened,
into the rose-garden.
T.S.Elloit (Four Quartets)
©1943, Houghton Mifflin Harcourt.

How passionate is one allowed to be about occupational group therapy? It is rather like being passionate about a group of roses. Your admiration of their collective beauty and fragrance encourages you to learn about roses and how to care for them. Your desire to grow them makes you carefully select the ones that will flourish in your garden and you position them with knowledge of their needs. Finally, you set about planting and looking after them. The nurtured product of your endeavours can be likened to the outcome from intervention by occupational group therapy which can be undertaken with groups of people from the young to the old, in different fields of health care.

There has been a remarkable growth and progression globally of occupational therapy into a scientific and meaningful profession with new models, techniques, equipment, research and evidence-based practice. However one is left with a sense that group-work in occupational therapy lags behind. There is some evidence-based research available worldwide on the subject, which will be addressed, but certainly not enough! This book attempts to address this subject by providing a practical guide and teaching manual for both under-graduate and postgraduate occupational therapy students. In this way they may increase their use of group work as a therapeutic intervention and draw inferences from their work which can be researched and published.

It is intended that this book has been written specifically for occupational group therapy intervention and some of the theory may be helpful to other professionals trained in groups.

The uniqueness of occupational group therapy relies on the fact that it is built on the theories of Yalom (1975), Moreno (1987) and Homans (1968) yet is well entrenched in occupational therapy philosophy and models from Canada, the United States, South Africa, the United Kingdom, Australia, etc. From this theoretical background the expertise to use activities of many kinds, which are the backbone of the occupational therapy profession, are woven into the dynamics of the group in a very effective manner.

The undergraduate occupational therapy curriculum covers client handling extensively as well as structuring and communicative skills, together with the therapeutic use of self. These are the ingredients for an effective group leader who excels in the functional and performance aspects that people need to develop.

Often we hear the words 'I don't feel confident and lack the experience to be a group leader'. Hopefully this is where this book comes in. Self-confidence is a quality that needs nurturing and practice within the occupational group therapy field. Make sure the essential learning is in place, attend experiential workshops for self-growth and use the guidelines and suggestions in this book to guide you.

The most effective group leaders are those who attend to the needs and feelings of group members in the present time and structure of the group, so that the stated goals are achieved (Health promotion Unit, NSW, Australia 1968). Choose your place and your clients, feed them and nurture them to the best of your ability and watch them grow.

You can walk down the passage of occupational group therapy, open the door, and admire your strongly growing, fragrant roses!

This book is being published in the midst of one of the most difficult times in the history of the world – the Covid 19 pandemic! However this does not change the fact that people still suffer from psychiatric, mental and psychological problems. In fact it exacerbates the problem. Occupation becomes paramount, especially during the lock-down and the World

Federation of Occupational Therapists (WFOT), and many countries and many countries have addressed this concept bringing occupational therapy to the forefront as an essential profession. As far as group work is concerned, it is clearly difficult to undertake group therapy whilst group members have to keep at a distance from one another and wear masks, but it is possible. Intervention is clearly compromised.

I wish to thank all occupational therapists who have persevered during this time and also my husband Michael who is a great support and experienced editor.

Foreword

Sharon Brintnell

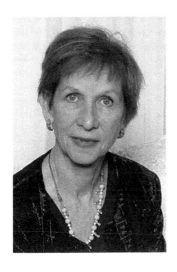

Rosemary Crouch and I met when we worked on many World Federation of Occupational Therapy (WFOT) initiatives such as the Education Committee. We met frequently at WFOT conferences and council meetings all over the world. In Ottawa in 1998 she became a Vice President of WFOT and I was Vice President (finance). Through our shared interests in education, mental health and psychiatry, as well as the global development of the occupational therapy profession, we became very close friends and always travelled in the countries where our meetings took place for a week or two together afterwards. Many happy times were had also with our respective husbands in South Africa, touring the wonderful game parks.

Throughout the many years of my knowing Rosemary, her passion has never waned from promoting excellence in occupational therapy education particularly in Africa and interventions for persons with mental illness. She also is recognised as an expert clinician in mental health and psychiatry. I have marvelled at and admired her energy and work ethic in leadership positions across academic, practice and regulatory domains ultimately in service to the public. Rosemary's influence remains on the curricular development of occupational therapy academic programmes in Tanzania, Uganda, Mauritius and Pakistan. Her mentorship in practice and writing has expanded the opportunities of many South African and other occupational therapists in sub-Saharan Africa to share their knowledge and expertise. By authoring a chapter in one of the two texts she edited solely or the four she co-edited with Vivyan Alers, these writers informed the world of the practice and research advancement in mental health occupational therapy and an African perspective on practice. The Crouch Bursary Fund was set up by Rosemary with the assistance of Vivyan to support the advancement and research of occupational therapy in psychiatric and mental health fields. Its funding comes from the royalties of their texts. Rosemary's encouragement and participatory manner in teaching has had an indelible effect on practitioners, undergraduates and postgraduate students.

Writing a forward for a new text is not an opportunity frequently offered, let alone to me. Rosemary Crouch is an extraordinary individual whose concern, dedication and efforts to the further development of the occupational therapy profession in Africa and the world have been reflected throughout her entire career. It is particularly evident through her promotion of knowledge dissemination through writing and taking on the authorship of this new book.

Occupational Group Therapy (OGT) is dedicated to Rosemary's dear friend and past collaborator, Vivyan Alers. The text is an advancement on group work, taking its core from emotional intensity awareness and occupational science writing. Though the text is now authored by Rosemary, its genesis arose from many discussions between these close friends in the garden and through observations at professional meetings in Africa and internationally. Finally, it was obvious that there was need to readdress action methods in different group experiences. A joint submission to the publisher for this initiative was accepted, but sadly Vivyan passed away suddenly in 2018 before her thoughts could be captured in her own words.

Throughout the chapters, readers will gain grounding in new ways of addressing familiar concerns as well as be challenged to expand their own offerings in occupational therapy groups. The collective experience of these two well-known and respected collators will be evident though expressed through a singular voice. There is no one more able to undertake the task than my dear friend Dr Rosemary Crouch.

It is my pleasure to invite you to explore this new exciting text with the view of first learning about and perhaps later experimenting with some of the techniques in your own work.

Professor Emerita Sharon Brintnell
Department of Occupational Therapy
Alberta University
Edmonton, Canada.

Introduction

Occupational therapists are experts in the use of occupation as both a means and an end to facilitating health, and promoting participation in meaningful life roles. Occupation thus forms an integral part of occupational therapy group work in all areas of occupational therapy practice. (OTASA 2014)

This book is specifically aimed at encouraging students and qualified occupational therapists who are using group work in their programmes to move to a higher and more dynamic level of therapeutic intervention, particularly in the use of occupation in their groups. For example, techniques such as assertiveness training and stress management can be mundane ordinary groups with the occupational therapist handing out notes at the end, or they can be experiential, meaningful, active techniques which have lasting effects on clients. Examples of these effects may be the ability to communicate more effectively or to develop interpersonal relationships, to relieve anxiety or even bring about changes in behaviour.

Working at a higher level of therapeutic intervention does not always require postgraduate training, but attending workshops and established professional groups can be very helpful in gaining confidence and skill. Not many of these opportunities are available and therefore this book is designed to possibly partly fill this gap, and encourage occupational therapists to employ a deeper level of working with groups and feel more confident about it.

Ideas and techniques are presented in each chapter, which lift the leadership and the group process to a higher level of intervention. Every occupational therapist interested in group work has the potential, backed up by their training, to use and develop their skills creatively and make a difference in their clients' lives. In this book the author is encouraging group leaders using this book to get involved in effective 'therapy' and design group experiences for their clients which will allow them to work on themselves.

This book does not address the dynamics of group work separately as they should have been entrenched in the study of group work at an undergraduate level. Dynamics are however woven into the techniques described.

It is also important to note that the author has not included material on groups with children. It is however recommended that the reader refer to the book 'Occupational Therapy in Psychiatry and Mental Health' Fifth Edition, Edited by Rosemary Crouch and Vivyan Alers in 2014 and published by Wiley and Blackwell in London.

In Part three of this book there are excellent chapters which refer to group work with children. The chapter 'Interdisciplinary Group Therapy with Children' by Marita Rademeyer and Diedre Niehaus is particularly recommended.

The author would like to acknowledge a significant contribution to this book by a very revered colleague and friend, Louise Fouché who has made a real change to the way occupational therapists in South Africa think and practise their profession as regards occupational group therapy. Her contribution to the training of occupational therapy students and graduates has been significant. She has also contributed to the statements made by the Occupational Therapy Association of South Africa (OTASA).

It should be noted that some of the concepts discussed by Louise as part of her specific model of group work, the Occupational Therapy Interactive Group Model (OTIGM) will be discussed again in various contexts in other chapters. The purpose is to consolidate the reader's understanding of the concepts within different occupational therapy interventions.

The author would also like to mention Dr Enos Romano who has also generously shared his research in occupational group therapy with the author for inclusion in the research chapter of this book. It is very valuable and highly recommended for occupational therapists to read his published articles in the journals as referenced.

The first section of the book deals with the theoretical underpinning of occupational group therapy, and the second part gives practical advice on certain well-used group techniques in the profession of occupational therapy. It is hoped that the addendums will be widely used by occupational group therapists in the field. The author acknowledges that Appendix A is colloquial in nature as the stress programmes that were specifically developed for an African rural environment. It is hoped that the reader can change them to suit the environment in which she/he is working. The actual programmes have been proved to be sound by scientific research.

THE THEORETICAL BACKGROUND

CHAPTER 1

Frames of Reference Relevant to Occupational Group Therapy and the Classification of Groups

1.1 FRAMES OF REFERENCE

What is a group? 'A small group is a collection of individuals who influence one another, derive some satisfaction from maintaining membership in the group, interact for some purpose, assume special roles, are dependent on one another and communicate face to face' (Tubbs 1978).

Borg and Bruce (1991) intimated that group work is an established treatment medium within occupational therapy. Group work has provided a focus for therapeutic intervention and broadly the aims are as follows:

- To develop a milieu where clients feel accepted and that they belong.
- Facilitation of sharing of ideas, emotions and problems.
- Influence on the changing of attitudes.
- Development of identity, confidence and self-esteem.
- Stimulation of motivation to carry out a task.
- Conflict resolution.
- Effective resource utilisation.
- Cost-effectiveness.

At the very beginning of the development of the profession of occupational therapy Anne Mosey put together some exciting concepts such as 'A group is more than a collection of individuals. Members of a group are bonded together by their group identity and shared purposes which will be realised by interacting and working together' (Mosey 1973).

Why Groups? What is it that actually makes group therapy an occupational therapists' choice of intervention when there are other methods available? Does one look at personal preference, or suitability in a particular clinical area which is related to curative factors for particular clients? It has to be a combination of both. 'We use groups because they are a naturally occurring phenomenon, which are known to have good and bad effects on people' Bundey et al. (1984). Fouché (2020) describes a group as part of a microcosm and states that 'The way you interact with others in the outside world will be the same way in which you will act and treat others in the group' (p. 14, Chapter 4). She also states that 'groups present a small society and have the same ingredients as any community'.

What are the curative factors? These are the specific aspects of groups that make them therapeutic and conducive to good health. Fouché in 2020 stated that 'As occupational therapists, we are goal-directed and therefore need to select appropriate curative factors which we would like to facilitate within each group' (See Chapter 4).

Theorists such as Yalom (1975) and Rogers (1961) have laid down the basic premises of the curative factors which are to be found within the processes of the group. Curative factors are strongly related to the dynamics of a group; for example cohesiveness, a basic dynamic which is essential to any group work, is the curative factor which allows members to be understood and feel safe. They also feel they are of value to the group.

Other curative factors are well defined by Yalom (1975) and include:

Instillation of hope.

Universality.

Imparting of information.

Altruism.

The recapitulation of the primary family.

Developing socialisation techniques.

Existential factors.

Imitative behaviour.

Group cohesiveness.

Interpersonal learning.

Catharsis.

Reflective appreciation.

These important factors are brought about mostly, but not entirely by the group leader's style and skill. All groups have to have a leader, which is described in this literature as the occupational therapist, but when working in a transdisciplinary setting may be another professional or a family member or layperson. It will depend on the setting.

Leaderless groups in any setting can become very destructive particularly in a clinical setting. Group members struggle to take over the group causing friction and conflict. It is very difficult to reach treatment goals. The dynamics of groups tell us that there is always a natural leader of any group of people but as occupational therapists, who are well trained in group work, we must be sure that the natural leader is the right person before allowing him/her to lead the group. They must be able to bring about the curative factors as described by Yalom.

1.2   CLASSIFICATION OF GROUPS AND TYPES OF OCCUPATIONAL GROUP THERAPY: DEFINING THE SCOPE OF OCCUPATIONAL GROUP THERAPY ACCORDING TO THE LEVEL OF EMOTIONAL INTENSITY

All types of occupational group therapy, from the simplest ADL (Activities of Daily Living) group to the more dynamic groups like psychodrama and assertiveness training are considered to be therapy. Linda Finlay (2002) states that: 'A classification of groups should not be interpreted rigidly. Any activity can be designed to fit along the continuum of task-social-communication-psychotherapy. In fact, all the elements may be on offer in any one group but shift according to what the group is doing and group member's responses' (Figure 1.1).

Model 1.1 is based on Finlay's model in Creek (2002, p. 246). Finlay addresses the approaches to group work in occupational therapy as:

- Skills-focused groups.
- Occupational behaviour groups.
- Cognitive behavioural groups.
- Psychodynamic creative therapy groups (Finlay in Creek 2002).

In the Position Statement on therapeutic group work in occupational therapy, the Occupational Therapy Association of South Africa (OTASA) states that 'Group work should address dysfunctional occupational performance area(s). In a mental health-care setting, social participation is often problematic, impacting occupational performance areas such as play, schooling and work.

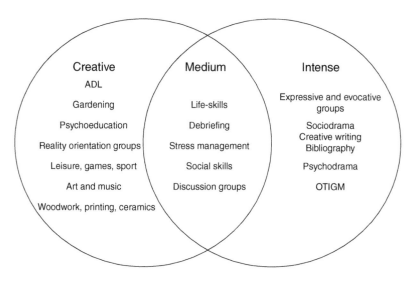

FIGURE 1.1   Diagram depicting the emotional categories of occupational group therapy. *Source*: Crouch and Fouché 2018.

The occupational therapist facilitates the group in such a way that each group member's poor social skills and impaired ability to build healthy interpersonal relationships i.e. social participation are addressed irrespective of the theme that is presented. Social skills are practised when interaction is actively facilitated within the group context' (OTASA 2014).

Types of groups:

- Groups to facilitate psychosocial adjustment to disability/illness.
- Education groups.
- Team-building groups.
- Exercise groups.
- Skills training groups.
- Group empowerment.

Functional Group Categories are also described by Howe and Schwartzberg in 1986. This progression shows the increase of emotional involvement on behalf of the group member. The categories are as follows:

- Activity groups:

  These are groups where members are involved in a common activity and are directed towards learning and maintaining occupational performance. This is explained in detail in Chapter 14.

- Intrapsychic groups:

  These are groups which deal with the insight into processes and conflicts that can occur within an individual. Psychodrama is a typical intrapsychic group and is explained in detail in Chapter 11.

- Social Systems groups:

  These are groups which follow the Systems Theory developed by Lewin (1951). They are aimed at increasing the interaction of participants.

- Growth groups:

  Growth Groups are generally aimed at increasing members' sensitivity to feelings or enhancing members 'ability to help them through the power of the group'. Howe and Schwartzberg (1986, p. 31).They are aimed at personal growth through action-orientated experiences. Growth groups are based on the principles of humanistic and existential philosophy and psychology that seek to fulfil the potential inherent in each person. These principles are explained in the writing of Rogers (1961), Shutz (1967), Perls et al. (1971) and Maslow (1962). Groups such as psychodrama, role-play and assertiveness training fall into this category.

Finlay succinctly describes the difference between group work and individual therapy. She states that 'both have their values for particular people, times and situations' (Finlay in Creek 2002, p. 249). She further states that 'Group work will be an appropriate choice of treatment if the patient or client:

- has the skills and awareness to interact and share with others in a group

- has problems related to social interaction and relationships
- feels isolated and is without others to offer support or constructive advice
- is threatened by the intensity or intimacy of one-to-one work'.

Groups falling out of the occupational therapy scope in South Africa but in which occupational therapists may be involved are as follows:

- Family Therapy groups.
- Social work groups.
- Psychotherapy groups.
- Art, music, drama and movement therapy groups.
- Marriage counselling groups.
- Teaching groups.

It should be noted by the reader that the above group techniques require further training which is not allowed for occupational therapists to perform in some countries.

CHAPTER 2

Research in Occupational Group Therapy

Research on the outcomes of intervention has become very important in countries such as South Africa where clients from the middle economic sector are supported by medical insurance/aid systems. Effectiveness of different techniques, time values, curative factors and analysis of quantitative and qualitative data are only some of the outcomes that need to be researched.

This is not the only reason, because in the broader urban and rural communities the accountability of the profession of occupational therapy depends on researched interventions which will be effective, economic and culturally suitable. Within the profession, occupational therapists need to make informed choices as to the type of intervention that is suitably employed. They need to be well informed and skilled to use group work within the economic environment and this depends to an extent on the research that has been undertaken on the subject. 'Research, therefore, is about understanding our world and the specific concepts in which we work. It is also about identifying limits and looking for alternative theories or approaches'. These are wise words from Jennifer Creek (2002, p. 54).

Occupational Group Therapy, First Edition. Rosemary Crouch.
© 2021 John Wiley & Sons Ltd. Published 2021 by John Wiley & Sons Ltd.

The World Health Organisation (WHO) stated in 2004 that 'Occupational therapists need to be able to demonstrate that therapeutic interventions are clinically effective so that the finite resources available can be used to deliver the best possible outcomes for the population served'. Ramano et al. states in his publication in 2018 that 'scientific rigor is required in occupational therapy research that supports the practice of activity-based groups for promoting social functioning' (p. 2).

In 1993 Finlay (in Creek 2002) stated that 'a lot of research on groups has been done, but findings are often contradictory and diversity of groups and outcomes studied can be confusing. Moreover, little of the research is related directly to occupational therapy practice'. (p. 205). There has been research into the comparison of individual activities to group work as well as freedom of choice in group activities by clients by Henry, Nelson and Duncombe in 1984. The results revealed that members should be involved in the choice and adaptation of group activities. Also in 1984 Kramer, Nelson and Duncombe studied the outcome of presenting three different types of activity to chronic psychiatric patients. They found differences in affective meaning. There have been a couple of descriptive studies undertaken which have not revealed a lot of significance.

Catherine Beynon-Pindar (2017) included an interesting chapter on group work in occupational therapy in her book 'Occupational Therapy Evidence in Practice for Mental Health'. She describes 'an intensive group programme to explore occupation-centred, evidence based approaches to group work practice in a residential setting' (p. 1, chapter 4). The population described consists of women with a variety of self-defeating behaviours, eating disorders and dissociation. She confirms that occupational group therapy is a core skill of the profession.

Crouch (1987) undertook a quantitative study which compared the effectiveness of certain occupational therapeutic group techniques in the assessment of acutely disturbed adult psychiatric patients. The objectives were to compare the evaluation/assessment of a psychiatric patient based on group observations with those assessments based on individual observations made by other members of the psychiatric team over a longer period of time. She also set out to validate the role of the occupational therapist in the use of group techniques for assessment purposes. The two types of groups used in the research were art groups and discussion groups. The occupational group therapy short-term assessments of the group members compared favourably with those assessments made by other team members over a longer period. It was found that the assessments made by the occupational therapist are a reliable contribution to the team evaluation of the patient and in a shorter period (Figure 2.1).

In more than a decade, the situation has changed considerably and there is some sound research on group work in occupational therapy emerging from all over the world.

In 2007 Crouch and Mogotsi undertook a research project in the psychiatric department of Johannesburg hospital. They assessed the efficacy of group writing in improving occupational performance, thereby enhancing employment possibilities and sustainability in

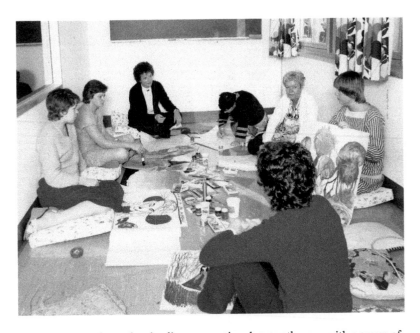

FIGURE 2.1   The author leading occupational group therapy with a group of patients in an acute psychiatric unit.

persons with bipolar affective disorder. The study took place over eight sessions using an experimental and control group. It was a longitudinal study and the results from the Canadian Occupational Performance Measure (COPM) showed a significant improvement in occupational performance in participants over a period of time.

Ramano and de Beer (2017) carried out an intensive and comprehensive research study on the improvement of social functioning of individuals with major depressive disorder (MDD). He compared the results of two occupational therapy group programmes over a period of four months. The study included 100 participants.

The outcome of Ramano's and de Beer (2017) research is that 'The therapeutic use of tangible activities and participants' social interaction in occupational therapy groups, are found to be curative and appropriate in reducing symptoms and improving functioning of patients with MDD since it enhanced their well-being' (p. 133). Ramano succeeded in isolating important symptoms of MDD such as lack of interest in everyday activities, tiredness and lack of energy, suicidal ideation, hopelessness, lack of concentration, etc. and through both quantitative and qualitative methods was able to conclude with significant results in the improvement of patients suffering from MDD.

In 2008 Crouch undertook intensive research into the use of stress management groups in the rural community in South Africa. This will be discussed further in Chapter 13.

In 2014 Casteleijn undertook doctorial research to establish that the sequential levels of creative ability according to DuToit (2009) measures increasing amounts of creative ability. The tool she developed is called the Activity Participation Outcome Measure (APOM). This outstanding research statistically confirms that 'the levels of creative ability exist and that the levels resemble the characteristics of an interval scale of measurement' (p. 181). This important finding is indeed very relevant to occupational group therapy and is being used in the measurement of outcomes regarding the performance of group members.

Included in Casteleijn's (2014) study is the Creative Participation Assessment Tool (CPA) which is a descriptive tool developed by van der Reyden in 2002 and has been used by occupational therapists and students to assess creative ability of participants in groups and individually. In 2002 Casteleijn and Smit adapted the CPA and established that it is valid and reliable.

Mona Eklund well-known occupational therapist in Scandinavia, published a paper on the Wile Online Library in April 2006 entitled 'Therapeutic Factors in Occupational Group Therapy identified by patients discharged from a Psychiatric Day Centre and their significant others'. She found that the most important factors of the group dimension were group interaction, talking in a group and the therapist's attitude and behaviour.

In 2019 Christopher undertook research into occupational therapy groups as a vehicle to address interpersonal relationship problems. Their study was aimed at the mental health care users' perceptions. This is a qualitative study where 11 groups specifically directed at interpersonal relationships were carried out. This study has specific reference to the content of this book and many of the chapters relate to occupational group therapy. The authors discuss how group members experienced a 'downward spiral' in interpersonal relationships supposedly caused by their mental illness. 'During group therapy, this downward cycle appeared to start to reverse, as the participant received acceptance, authentic support, and social connection. This seemed to have provided a safe place to practices social skills and as a result strengthen self-esteem, and positive relationships, leading to a greater level of acceptance and mental health' (in Radnitz et al. 2019, p. 8.). This article is highly recommended.

Very little research is to be found on group work with the physically disabled. Mehdizadeh et al. (2017) published an excellent research paper on stroke survivors and the effect of group-based occupational therapy on performance and satisfaction. Their results show a significant change and improvement in ADL performance but unfortunately they do not state the effect that working in a group had on the clients.

CHAPTER 3

Models of Occupational Therapy Relevant to Occupational Group Therapy

3.1 THE FUNCTIONAL GROUP MODEL

This model was developed a long time ago by Howe and Schwartzberg (1986) but has some relevance to modern-day occupational group therapy. The Functional Group Model is an occupational therapy approach to group work. Howe and Schwartzberg (1986) make three statements about the Functional orientation of the functional group:

- 'Functional groups provide a place for members to function in the reality of the present and to practice skills in decision making, judgment, and perception, as well as in areas of specific deficits.

- Functional groups are concerned with elements of performance as well as types of performance, such as work, play, and self- maintenance.
- Functional groups seek to build group cohesiveness; a certain degree of cohesiveness is necessary to achieve functional goals' (p. 99).

The reader will note that these statements are very much in line with modern thinking on occupational group therapy as discussed by Louise Fouché (in Chapter 4) and the Model of Occupational Performance (Law et al. 1994).

What is meant by a 'Functional Group' The aim of a Functional Group is for group members to take part in purposeful active participation. They are involved in a meaningful product which will bring about learning and skills and social interaction, address emotional needs, build on strengths and all of this will take place in the 'here-and-now' (Moreno 1975). It will be experiential in nature and spontaneous action should take place.

Howe and Schwartzberg (1986) state that 'The process of establishing norms in a group helps the group interact in the "here and now" context because norms refer to immediate concerns'. They stress the importance of the genuine exploration of conflicts and problems which are shared by the group. The importance of spontaneity, as stressed by Moreno in 1975, brings about trust in the group which is essential in the early development of the group. This is known as the formative stage of a group and is defined by a number of theorists e.g. Tubbs and Moss (1981). The development stage builds on the formative stage. The occupational group therapist will adapt the task to meet the development of the group as explained clearly by Louise Fouché (2020). Once the group members have worked out conflict issues, tested the safety of the group and any power struggles etc. they can continue into the "Work phase".

3.2   THE VdTMOCA MODEL

Formal research has been undertaken in South Africa on a Model of Occupational Therapy called the VdTMoCA (the Vona duToit Model of Creative Ability).This model does not specifically address a model of group work but is very relevant to patients and clients treated by occupational therapists in groups. According to van der Reyden and Sherwood (2019) 'The VdTMoCA provides a theoretical framework for understanding people and their activity participation in terms of creative ability, which has a specific meaning in this model' (p.60).

Much emphasis is placed today on the diligent assessment of patients/clients who are selected to participate in a group as part of their therapy, particularly in occupational therapy. It is extremely important for patients/clients to derive the maximum benefit from their group therapy by being chosen to be in a group with other people who actively participate in their lives at the same, or similar, level of creative ability.

Meaningful activity participation is perhaps the most important concept in this theory which directly relates to occupational group therapy. Du Toit states in 1962 that 'It is thus through activity participation that there is the experience of living, the potential for growth, and realisation of one's capabilities and potential i.e. realisation of one's self' (p. 65).

De Witt and Sherwood (2019) in their discussion of du Toit's Model mention situations in relation to behaviours, and adherence to various norms related to relational engagement in group activities. As noted by Louise Fouché in her work, a group provides an excellent opportunity for the occupational therapists to observe how group members relate to each other. De Witt and Sherwood (2019) noted that 'relational contact with others can be observed through the person's ability to recognise others and engage with them in a socially appropriate manner through greetings, taking of instruction or directions, sharing of tools, materials and space' (p. 170).

It is acknowledged that there are other factors that are important too in selecting members of a group such as age and diagnosis. These are factors that are interwoven into creative ability but can also stand alone, e.g. selecting an homogeneous group of elderly, depressed women, although functioning on the same level of creative ability, will lead to disaster. There will be little motivation and could lead to an increase in depression. It is generally acknowledged by group therapists that groups should be heterogeneous.

3.3   THE CANADIAN MODEL OF OCCUPATIONAL PERFORMANCE (CMOP)

This model which was developed in 1991 is widely used throughout the world. It defines the three basic areas of occupational performance, i.e. self-care, productivity and leisure. See Figure 3.1 below.

The Canadian Occupational Performance Measure (COPM) based on the CMOP was developed as 'an individualised measure of a client's self-perception in occupational performance, and is designed to be used in client-centred occupational therapy practice'. (Law et al. 1994).

No particular mention is made of the use of group work specifically because the model applies to most types of occupational therapy intervention. It is well known and has been used in many research projects, including Crouch and Mogotsi (2007) who used occupational group therapy and the COPM successfully in assessing performance in persons with bipolar disorders. In most cases such as this, the assessment is carried out initially in order to identify problem areas

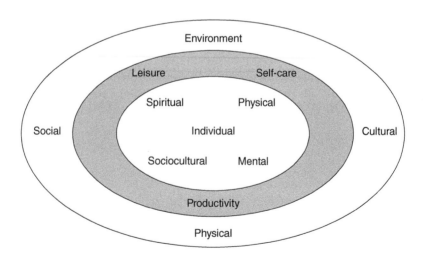

FIGURE 3.1   The Canadian Model of Occupational Performance.

of occupational performance in the members of the group. The whole group can then establish what the goals of the group will be. After a period, the assessment is used again by group members to see if there has been a change in occupational performance and how satisfied group members are with the changes.

In the COPM, the client is required to assess him/herself. The relevance of using this assessment with clients taking part in occupational group therapy is the unique fact that the assessment comprises the client's own assessment of his/her performance in the group itself and his/her satisfaction with the performance in the group. Consequently there are two types of scores: performance and satisfaction. 'Occupational performance is an experienced phenomenon rather than an observed phenomenon' (Law et al. 1994, p. 5).

As indicated, the model also provides an opportunity for reassessment. 'At an appropriate interval following the initial assessment, a reassessment takes place. The time interval is variable and depends on the client's and therapist's judgement, but it is suggested that an expected date of reassessment be agreed upon before intervention begins' (Law et al. 1994, p. 44).

3.4   THE MODEL OF HUMAN OCCUPATION (MOHO)

This model by Gary Kielhofner was developed in 1980 and the latest publication was 2002. The model identifies three constructs namely person, environment and occupational performance, all of which are basic concepts relevant to occupational group therapy. He emphasises occupational participation which is described as occupational identity, occupational adaptation and occupational competence which are all vitally important when participating as a member of a group. One important factor in this model is his interpretation of 'meaning' as being a determining factor in occupational engagement, a factor essential to participation in occupational group therapy. If a group member feels that group work has meaning for him/her it may result in feelings of competence, confidence and security as regards their abilities. 'An assumption underlying the MOHO is that by engaging in occupation, humans learn values and skills and develop interests, a sense of self-confidence and competence' (Townsend and Polatajko 2007, p. 60). All of these factors are basic and extremely relevant to occupational group therapy.

CHAPTER 4

The Occupational Therapy Interactive Group Model (OTIGM): Reconnecting to Me Through My Interaction with You in the "Here and Now"

Louise Fouché

No man is an island. Human beings were created to be social beings. In other words, human beings need people and healthy relationship to be mentally healthy, to be functional optimally and to thrive in all occupational performance areas. People cannot lead quality lives without having others with which to share their life. The old English proverb 'a sorrow shared, is a sorrow halved and a joy shared, is a joy doubled' has deep wisdom.

Occupational Group Therapy, First Edition. Rosemary Crouch.
© 2021 John Wiley & Sons Ltd. Published 2021 by John Wiley & Sons Ltd.

One of the prominent problems of all clients that approach an occupational therapist for intervention, is that due to their illness/disorder/disability, they have withdrawn from previous relationships, or they have shut others out or they have never been able to form good interpersonal relationships. Irrespective of the field of occupational therapy, interpersonal relationship, or as the American Practice Framework defines it, social participation, should be assessed and if indicated, addressed in therapy.

Group therapy or group work, or as South African occupational therapists have defined it, occupational group therapy, still remains one of the most effective techniques in addressing problem areas with the occupational performance area of social participation.

This chapter sets out to describe an occupational group therapy model, known as the Occupational Therapy Interactive Group Model (OTIGM). This model was designed and developed in South Africa in the mid-1980s by an occupational therapist, M de Beer and a psychologist, C Vorster. The chapter sets out a brief history of the model, the basic principles of the model, effective techniques to implement, group procedures to follow and will end with examples of group narratives in understanding the therapeutic value of the model. The model has developed and grown over the years, and hybrids have formed, where different occupational therapists emphasise slightly different aspects of the model. However this chapter will provide a good overview of the model, keeping it simplistic for those who are unfamiliar with it.

4.1   A BRIEF HISTORY

Dr Marianne de Beer was lecturing at the University of Pretoria in the early 1980, and recalls that she felt unprepared and not confident in her knowledge or skills of groups to teach group work to the occupational therapy students. De Beer was promised that resources would be made available in her quest to improve her knowledge and skills in group work. She then visited all the occupational therapists who had become well known for their group skills across South Africa, people like Rosemary Crouch, Dain van der Reyden,

Madeleine Duncan. She observed them leading groups and interviewed them. De Beer explained that she observed excellent, effective therapy, and when she questioned them, their answers were based on their therapeutic experiences, excellent clinical reasoning and instinct as occupational group therapists. Each occupational therapist presented groups differently and there did not seem to be one way to present groups which could be used to extrapolate a unifying theory. De Beer realised that was not enough to provide guidelines or training for occupational therapy students, who often had neither the experience nor the natural instincts within groups.

De Beer then approached Professor Vorster, who was lecturing at the Department of Psychology at the University of Pretoria at the time. She joined his group therapy sessions participating and spending time immersing herself in the theory and application. Vorster supported Yalom's perspective of group therapy and taught his students the Group Psychotherapy principles. However, in the pure form these principles are not within the occupational therapy scope of practice as defined by the Occupational Therapy Board at the Health Professionals Council of South Africa. At this point Vorster and de Beer collaborated and developed the Occupational Therapy Interactive Group Model (OTIGM), specifically designed for occupational therapists. This model has been used since the mid-1980s to train students at the Medical University of South Africa (Medunsa) and at the University of Pretoria and later for under- and postgraduate students at the University of the Witwatersrand. The model has grown since then and although occupational therapists may emphasise different aspects of the model within their clinical application, they remain true to the core of the model.

4.2 THE OCCUPATIONAL THERAPY INTERACTIVE GROUP MODEL IN CONTEXT

There are numerous different approaches to group therapy. Each approach and theory has specific underlying assumptions on which the therapeutic intervention is based. Some examples are cognitive-behavioural groups, Rogerian groups, expressive groups,

Dialectic-Behavioural Therapy, etc. The Occupational Therapy Interactive Group Model follows a psychosocial approach.

The psychosocial approach emphasises the importance of people as social beings and the role interpersonal relationships have on mental health and well-being. Occupational therapists that strictly follow a Psychosocial: Interactive approach, take it one step further and believe that illness is rooted in poor relationships. Due to problems experienced within intimate or significant relationships, mental health care users develop unhealthy interpersonal patterns. This causes them to become overly anxious about forming relationships and they either withdraw or avoid others or continue unhealthy patterns. As they withdraw, they have fewer opportunities to keep their social skills intact and their social skills become neglected. This makes it even more difficult for them to form new and healthy interpersonal relationships. This lack of interpersonal relationships causes psychological discomfort which can culminate in a mental illness. In a nutshell one of the assumptions of the approach is that a break in relationships is the cause of mental illness and in order to improve mental health and well-being, interpersonal relationships need to be addressed.

If occupational therapists believe this premise and follow the Psychosocial: Interactive approach, it stands to reason that they would need to focus on the mental health care users' interpersonal relationships, his/her behaviour patterns and his/her poor social skills during treatment. If these are not pertinently addressed in therapy, the occupational therapist would merely be treating the mental health care user symptomatically which means the cause of the illness would be ignored, allowing the symptoms to return as soon as they become stressed or treatment is ended. The root cause (in terms of interpersonal relationships and social skills, i.e. occupational social participation) needs to be identified and treated in order for treatment to be effective and long-lasting. This is the theoretical foundation and premise on which the Occupational Therapy Interactive Group Model is based; only then can occupational group therapy become effective and life-changing.

In essence the Occupational Therapy Interactive Group Model focuses on training or changing social skills, focuses on forming healthy interpersonal relationships, all within the group context. The occupational therapist achieves this by facilitating interaction between the group participants. Through the interaction, cohesion, i.e. a sense of belonging and acceptance is facilitated that allows group members to feel safe enough to take risks. The risks can be: trying new behaviour patterns, new social skills and new ways of relating to other people within their group. Core to the model are principles of the 'here-and-now' (Moreno 1975), process illumination, selection of activity as a catalyst, and are all techniques used as a means to improve mental health care users' social skills and interpersonal relationships. The model moves away from didactic (or psycho-educational groups) and instead of talking about a subject like assertiveness (or conflict management or stress management), these skills are facilitated in the here-and-now, as and when a specific group member requires the skills within the group. Therefore, the model provides opportunities for group members to interact, to relate to each other, through the participation in carefully, selected activity(ies). Each group participant and the group collectively then reflect on the group members' experiences. They can reflect on their habits, behaviours, social skills, methods of relating to each other within the group as displayed during the specific activity. At times feedback is provided by fellow group members in order for the group member to develop insight as to the impact his/her skills and behaviour had on others in the group. New opportunities are facilitated in order to change these behaviours or practise the new skills, in the group, right here, right now.

Groups are a generic technique/medium/skill used by many professionals but occupational therapists all over the world should to be clear as to the unique contributions which they bring to groups used as intervention in treatment. They can incorporate their unique knowledge and skills with group work especially regarding occupational performance areas and activities/tasks analysis and selection. They have something exclusive and distinctly different to offer in comparison to other health care professionals.

4.3 THE 'HERE-AND-NOW'

Reference will continually be made to the 'here-and-now' concept. This concept is core to the OTIGM and was defined by Jacob Moreno (father of Psychodrama) in 1920 (see Chapter 11 on Psychodrama).

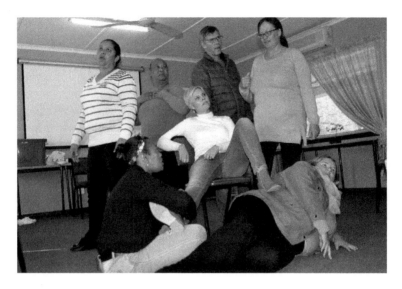

FIGURE 4.1   Psychodrama: building our community as a person (main activity).

Blatner (1973) intimated that speaking in the here-and-now tends to pull the group member 'into the interaction as if it were actually happening there for the first time' (p. 16).

What has occurred in the past cannot be changed and the future still needs to happen and both can be considered in the there-and-then. When group members focus on the past or future, the group becomes stuck and will automatically start to disengage and the interaction between group members decreases. The occupational therapist will sense that the group lacks energy and progress is slow. The feeling can be described as 'dragging' the group members along.

The here-and-now implies that the focus is on what is happening *now* within the group, right at this moment, *here* in this group. For example, if a group participant starts sharing about a past experience, the occupational therapist can say 'I wonder what bearing your sharing has on the group, at this moment'. The occupational therapist calls the group member's attention back to the group. Initially group members are taken back and will quickly deny it has relevance. With some encouragement, they will inevitably identify the link. For example, the occupational therapist brings the group back to the here-and-now, by rephrasing the comment: 'You explained how someone who was special to you dropped you. What relevance does that have on this group? Do you fear this group will drop you?' The occupational therapist can follow-up this question with different options. She/he can facilitate curative factors like universality (who else have been dropped? or who else feels afraid of being dropped by the group?) or interpersonal learning (does anyone want to give Ms K any feedback?). The occupational therapist can facilitate process illumination (what is your reaction to Ms K's statement?) or another here-and-now question (what do you need right now in this group to feel safer? Or who in this group, at this moment, do you feel is least likely to drop you?).

The essence of the here-and-now is to not focus on problems outside the group or past history, but to focus on what is happening in the group, at this moment, because changes can be facilitated in the here-and-now.

4.4 OCCUPATIONAL THERAPY INTERACTIVE GROUP MODEL'S CORE PRINCIPLES

What does an occupational therapist aim to facilitate within a group? What is he/she striving to achieve within a group? For example, ask the question: if a person in the group says 'I really find it difficult to deal with my stress and these methods just don't work for me?' What should the occupational therapist strive to achieve? How would she/he facilitate interaction with this statement? She could give more advice/ another technique or try to problem-solve the reason for the difficulty with a stress management method or try to find out where the difficulty comes from. Alternatively, the occupational therapist could ask other group members if they have similar experiences (universality). The choice the occupational therapist makes will depend on the overarching aim of occupational therapy groups, the principles followed and the theme of the group. The occupational therapist should be crystal clear on what she/he is trying to achieve, else the group can end up with group participants being passive and the occupational therapist is doing all the work with minimal impact and no change of behaviour.

Before continuing with the principles, it is important to distinguish between occupational therapy group work and occupational group therapy. Occupational therapy group work is where there are a number of mental health care users together in the same room, doing the same activity or task. They are each participating as individuals and it is much the same as individual therapy except that the group members do participate socially to some extent. For example, a craft group is occupational therapy within a group context when each patient is busy with his/her own craft activity, in their own world, with their own thoughts, only briefly aware of anyone else or occasional connecting with other group members. For low-level mental health care users particularly, there is value in this type of group work (see Chapter 14). However, the main purpose of occupational group therapy is to facilitate interaction between group members. In this way interpersonal relationships are actively formed and dynamics between group participants are facilitated to bring about insight and healing and an opportunity is provided to try and practise new social skills or behaviours. Interaction between the group participants is essential to their treatment and the outcomes obtained in occupational group therapy can in no way be obtained when seeing patients individually.

These two types of groups differ considerably in terms of time, energy and areas of concern which the occupational therapist would concentrate on and facilitate during the group. For example, a social skills group following a cognitive-behavioural approach would spend time and energy on group members learning a specific social skill such as initiating a conversation, so that at the end of the group session, the mental health care users are skilled in that particular social skill. On the other hand, in an occupational group therapy session time and energy will be spent with group participants actively participating in an activity and then facilitate feedback between group members about each person's social skills and the impact it has on others as experienced in the here-and-now, within this group activity. The occupational therapist will additionally create opportunities for group members to interact with each other by facilitating curative factors. This will be the ultimate goal throughout all the groups presented, irrespective of the theme or activity selected.

4.5   LEADING FROM BEHIND

A core concept of the OTIGM is that the occupational therapist is a facilitator over and above anything else. This means the occupational therapist is not a 'leader' as is commonly understood. There is a continuum where on the one hand group members are allowed to do anything they want, including having a friendly chit-chat group on the side, and on the other hand being told exactly what they have to do. Both these are not conducive to effective, therapeutic groups. Within the OTIGM, an appropriate metaphor for the occupational group therapist would be to 'lead like a sheep dog'. The sheep dog knows where the sheep need to go and allows them to walk ahead. When the sheep then start to stray too much to the left or right, the sheep dog gently brings them back on the path towards the kraal. There is therefore not an exact path the sheep follow every day. Sometimes they stray more to the left and other times more to the right, but they are headed in the right direction.

This implies that the occupational group therapist is open to the group members' needs and their process. They progress at their own pace. No group should be forced in any direction. The group follows their own process and only when they are on the 'wrong' path (or their interaction is none therapeutic) does the occupational group therapist refocus them or bring them back to the important issues. For example, the group members may try to avoid anger issues and then change the subject. The occupational group therapist points this out to the group and facilitates the here-and-now process: this constitutes both the experience and the illumination process.

It is important to remember that should the group arrive at a point where they can either focus on the specific theme selected by the occupational therapist prior to the session or deeper issues or needs that have arisen in the here-and-now within the group, it is imperative for the occupational therapist to follow the group process and explore the issues voiced by the group. The group will be more therapeutic as the group participants are addressing a specific need voiced by the group. Should the occupational therapist force the group members to remain with her/his preselected theme, she/he will notice that the group participant's energy levels will decrease and it will feel as if the group members are 'dragging their feet' because it is against the greatest need currently in the group. This could be compared to a person wanting to talk to their significant other about a pressing need and then being told 'Wait, I first want you to talk to my mother'. How present will that person be in the conversation about the mother?

If the occupational group therapist is not the leader but 'leads' from behind, what does that look like in practice? The occupational therapist creates opportunities for group members to express themselves and their needs. She/he provides opportunities for group members to explore different activities. The less structured the groups are and the more interaction is facilitated, the more the occupational therapist will become aware of the group's needs. By following the group procedures, the occupational therapist allows the group members a chance to indicate their needs during the bridging stage and allows the group members to freely choose whether to 'sign a contract' for the occupational therapist's specific preselected theme. It should not be a manipulative process by which she/he forces the selected theme onto the group. If she/he is truly open to their needs, effective therapy will take place.

The occupational therapist can also leave decisions for the group to make and incorporate choices on a daily basis. For example, 'How are you feeling as a group at this moment? We can continue with the theme on forgiveness I prepared for the group or we can address the issue of trust that we have just identified from the warm-up. What would you like to do?' Even though it may take some time for the group to reach consensus, it is important for the occupational therapist to be a facilitator and allow the group members to come to a decision. This process in itself should be closely observed by the occupational therapist as the process could have the potential to facilitate the here-and-now, especially if specific dynamics reoccur, e.g. Mrs J is a group member who always makes the decision for the group; is passive and then complains about the choice later.

This concept provides numerous opportunities for the group members to take responsibility for their own healing process. The group decides and the occupational therapist provides opportunities and activities to assist the group to reach their choices, dreams and healing. The occupational therapist no longer has to have the answers and fix problems or find the most effective way to deal with an awkward situation in the group. She/he will give it back to the group and ask them how they would like to continue. For example, 'I see there is an uncomfortable silence in the group. What is happening in the group at the moment? What would you like to do about it?' Group members often surprise the occupational therapist with their suggestions (often suggestions she/he has not even considered).

Here is an example to understand the concept: In a group, one group participant, Mrs R is disabled and in a wheel chair. The warm-up activity selected required physical activity. Mrs R was reluctant to participate and was encouraged by the occupational therapist to ask the group what they could suggest. In this particular group, two strong men in the group offered to hold up Mrs R and she agreed. After the warm-up, the group reflected about the situation and the two strong men thanked Mrs R for allowing her the opportunity to share their strength in service of the group (altruism). In turn Mrs R started to apologise to the group about her disability. The group members stopped her and provided empowering feedback saying any one of them could become disabled at any stage and there is no reason to apologise. This led to Mrs R becoming emotional (catharsis) and shared how she constantly felt guilty about her disability. Instead of the occupational therapist causing her to withdraw from the warm-up activity or changing the activity to suit Mrs R, so much healing took place because Mrs R engaged with the group and together, they found the solution that suited this group best. In the process Mrs R found a new perspective on her disability and was assisted to voice her needs.

4.6   GROUPS AS A 'MINI-SOCIETY'

Groups present a small society. Metaphorically, the group could be seen as a slice taken from society. It is made up of the same 'ingredients' as any community or society and has the same requirements as a society. The group is made up of different people from different cultures, with different opinions, different religious beliefs, different sexual orientation, different values and dreams, different socioeconomic status and from different ages. Within a group, each individual is required to interact with others in a manner that is respectful, truthful, etc. There are no different norms in the group than required by society for example to respect others, not interrupt others talking, to make eye contact, etc.

People tend to have specific views and prejudices around other people's 'otherness'. Human beings quickly label and place people in 'us' versus 'them' categories as this creates security and safety. However, at the same time it creates disregard for the 'them' and keeps people blind to the full truth of any situation. The therapeutic value of a group is that as in society that contains people with such a wide range of differences, people can sit in a group and truly listen to others and start to understand. Questions can be asked and prejudices confronted within the group. In a sense healing happens as the stereotype now becomes a person with a face, a name, with feelings and especially in a cohesive group, this person has been placed within an 'us'-context. This silently breaks downs the differences that divide society. Take Mrs R from the above example who was a wheelchair-bound group participant. The group members could ask Mrs R questions regarding living with disability to improve their understanding, but within each group session, there is a deeper understanding and empathy that merges at the group members become witnesses to Mrs R's difficulties. Even more important they share experiences of their shared humanness, that Mrs R is a person who laughs about the same things and was hurt by similar life situations.

(Fouché 2020)

Disability will no longer be a distant concept for each group member after they leave the group. Stereotypes of people with disability will have been irrevocably changed.

Additionally, as each group is a 'mini-society' and represents society as a whole, the very issues that the society is currently dealing with will be brought into the group space. A while back, South Africa highlighted gender-based violence. It was a big discussion point in schools, in workplaces, in businesses, in social media with constant Facebook sharing and tweets on the topic. Some felt men were not taking enough responsibility for fellow males to change their views and behaviour towards women. It was then not surprising when a male group participant, Mr F, was strongly confronted by female group members when he made a disparaging gender-stereotype joke during a group activity. This led to an intense discussion. Some group members vouched for Mr F's character saying he was gentle and kind and did not mean it and would never hurt a fly. One or two group members shared their life experiences of gender-based violence and explained how the comment made them feel. Mr F apologised saying that was not his intention at all, and continued how he felt judged and categorised just because he is a male. The occupational therapist allowed the discussion to continue so that both sides could be heard. At a later stage she/her asked the group 'what stance would the group like to take on this issue' and 'what does that mean for this group?' What behaviour or remarks are acceptable within your group?

Yalom (1975) states that groups are the most truthful place people will experience. It is not the occupational therapist's job to steer group members away from the difficult conversations. If these conversations are not held in a safe, cohesive group, where would be more suitable? This is the reason that the author developed occupational therapy group training in an organisation called OTGrow and their motto is 'Healing South Africa one group at a time'.

This group concept should encourage the occupational therapist to select more heterogeneous group members. The more diverse the group members are, the more diverse the opinions and thoughts are represented, the more conflict is likely, but also the greater the healing that occurs.

4.7   GROUPS AS PART OF A MICROCOSM

The way people interact with others in the world outside the group will be the same way in which they interact with others in the group. For example, if someone is a people-pleaser at his/her home or at work, it is assured he/she will be a people-pleaser within the group. It is logical because if he/she could change this behaviour or pattern, it would have already happened. However, this behaviour has become so much part of life over the past years that this behaviour is ingrained and automated. Mental health care users have become trapped by these behaviour patterns which cause them heartache and pain, but they are often unaware of their behaviour patterns and the impact they have on others.

During groups, using the here-and-now technique, the person is made aware of this behaviour by means of truthful feedback from the group members. To take the example of the people-pleaser, the other group members can explain to the person how the people-pleasing behaviour impacts them. '*I get fed-up when you are continuously trying to please others and I start to wonder who you really are. I want to get to know who you are; what your opinions are even though they may differ from mine. I don't want to have a friend that is a copy of me. But I never get the opportunity to get to know you because you spend so much time wanting to do what I want. Then I would rather try to make friends with someone else in the group*'. It is imperative that it is not left there, but that the group members are asked how they would suggest the person changes this behaviour. The more specific and practical the suggestion, the better. Most suggestions can be made on a basic verbal or nonverbal communication level. The change should be implemented within the group from then onwards. Another example is: There was a mental health care user in a group that used very sophisticated language when talking to the group members. This social skill, or rather her method of talking in the group, is the same manner in which she talks to people outside the group. During the group, it became obvious that she would talk a lot, but after she finished nobody would respond or comment on anything she said. There would be silence. She would then break the silence and explain herself all over again. When the group cohesion was strong enough, the occupational therapist facilitated feedback from the group members as to the impact that the sophisticated language had on them. A couple of group members explained that they often did not even understand what she was trying to say and they felt too dumb to ask. Once she realised it was her sophisticated language that shut others down, she started to practise talking in a manner that others could understand. The group agreed they would help her and every time they could not understand what she was saying in the group, they told her and she could practise talking more simplistically, right at that moment in the group. It was important to observe the aha moment she experienced, realising that people outside the group reacted the same way, and could understand why people started to avoid her. Now she had the knowledge and insight and was building up her social skill, specifically her verbal communication, to be able to better connect with people, especially within her work context.

Initially occupational therapists feel uncomfortable to facilitate truthful feedback. They are concerned that the feedback is harmful to the mental health care user. Yet surprisingly there are minimal times that a group participant outrightly rejects the feedback, especially if the cohesiveness in the group is strong. The majority of group participants experience relief and insight. They often say they have realised for a long time they are doing something wrong, but do not know what it is. Their maladaptive social skills have led to people outside in their community to avoid them or unnecessarily confront them which leaves them feeling rejected or isolated. The majority of the time the feedback can be broken down into verbal and nonverbal communication aspects, which firstly can be rectified with practice and secondly indicates that it is not the person themselves that is rejected, but their poor social skill. However, it is imperative that there is strong cohesive group before the occupational therapist facilitates feedback. The group participant must feel that sense of acceptance and belonging in the group, before feedback is given.

The reason that this principle is healing is because people will automatically play out their own pathology, as the group is a part of the microcosm. This allows the occupational therapist to directly treat social participation elements within the group, knowing that the maladaptive behaviour patterns or poor social skills displayed in the group are the very same ones the person is using outside. In-depth assessment of each mental health care user's social participation is no longer as imperative; in most cases, mental health care users lack insight into their poor social skills and maladaptive behaviour. Placing them within a group context and observing them during group activities becomes the most reliable assessment. Mental health care users who are dominating outside will be dominating in the group. Those that manipulate others outside will manipulate their fellow group members.

4.8   CHANGES THAT OCCUR IN THE GROUP, ARE TAKEN BACK TO SOCIETY

Any changes that occur within the group will be taken back by the mental health care user to their home, work and community. Any prejudice or paradigm that was questioned will bring change within the mental health care user. When this experience is accompanied with a strong emotional experience, the impact for change is greater. Similarly any feedback from fellow group members has a greater influence, due to the deep connections received formed within a cohesive group. This is the reason that the occupational therapist should focus on cohesiveness from the first group session.

In practice, the occupational therapist strives to bring about change within the group context. The idea of psycho-education group where topics are discussed and then attendees are expected to change their behaviour and thoughts is not realistic. The occupational therapist focuses on creating opportunities for:

(i) Uncomfortable discussions where group members are encouraged to truthfully voice their opinions and thoughts.

(ii) Giving feedback to group members specifically on the manner in which their behaviour or prejudice or poor social skills impact people in the group.

(iii) Specific suggestions to change poor social skills.

(iv) Providing opportunities to practise the new social skill or new behaviour pattern.

(v) Facilitating curative factors.

For example, if there is a group member who finds it particularly difficult to connect to people in the group and she/he can be asked pertinently, 'What can you do, right here and now, in the group to take the first step to connect to your group members?' Wait for the suggestion to come from the person. If they are struggling, pose the question to the group. As occupational therapists, with the skills of activity analysis, one or two actual activities can be provided as options in which this specific element is incorporated. For example, one group participant said she wanted to be physically connected to group members, she wanted to stand inside a circle made by the group members and that group members should reach out and touch her. The occupational therapist used this as a basis of an activity where each group member, one-by-one, verbalised to the group participant in the way they felt specifically connected to her and then place their hands on her. After the activity, the occupational therapist facilitated reflections with regard to every one's experience of the activity. The example serves to explain the importance of challenging the group participant to take the first step to bring about change within the group. Once the person returns home, it is not as daunting to connect to others within her own community – after all she had already taken the first step in the group. The stronger the cohesion, the braver group members become in taking risks, making suggestions and taking first steps.

4.9 THE WHOLE IS GREATER THAN THE SUM OF THE PARTS

The scientific principle of 'whole is the greater than the sum of the parts' applies particularly to occupational group therapy. If seven different individuals are placed in the group, the interaction and dynamics that develop will be different than if each person was seen separately using the same activity and then placed all end products together. Another scenario, if these seven people were placed within a group, but not provided opportunities to interact or work together, the end products will be similar to their individual end products with maybe one or two small differences brought about by seeing someone else's work and then adjusting their own.

If seven people are placed in a group, each bringing in their own flavour, own strengths and weaknesses, and then asked to create something together, the group becomes a melting pot of everyone's flavour, strength and weakness, which accumulatively or collectively will become this group's flavour, strength and weaknesses. The reason is that each individual is expected to bring of themselves to ensure the group can function as a group. Certain parts of each person will need to be compromised for the greater good of the group. Yet this does not diminish the group in any way but actually creates a greater group, a greater whole.

Certain norms, both covert and overt, are established which all group members start to conform, e.g. one person may be shy and an introvert and if seen individually would wait for the occupational therapist to direct the questions and encourage participation. However, place this person in a group with more extroverted participants and the group may prescribe a norm for everyone to participate in all the activities. The shy patient now has a choice, either he/she needs to comply with the norm and put effort into participating in order to be part of the group or he/she can disagree and risk being confronted or rejected by the group. His/her behaviour alone may change and it would require that more aspects of himself/herself are brought to the group. By placing people together in a group, the norms (overt and covert), the connections, attractions and repulsions between certain group members, the relationships formed, the expectations, etc. add so many facets to the group.

The implications for the occupational therapist in practice is to allow each group to form and progress at their own pace and to select numerous tasks/activities that provide an opportunity for the group to work together. For example, it is more effective to ask a group to design their own graffiti wall, than giving each person a coloured pen and asking them to write on a communal graffiti wall. The occupational therapist should provide opportunities for group choices and allow time afterwards to reflect on the dynamics and process in making decisions. The occupational therapist can speed up the process by taking herself/himself out of the activity/task and the group members are then left to talk with each other instead of speaking to him/her as their default mode. In group training workshops, there is an expectation that group members take tea and lunch together. Care should be taken not to allow group participants to leave or to be taken out of the group by other multidisciplinary team members as that keeps changing the dynamics with a group and creates insecurity and disequilibrium. Closed groups are more effective because the 'whole' formed by the group, with specific dynamics and identify forms strong cohesive groups.

4.10   GROUPS FORM THEIR OWN IDENTITY

All groups develop an identity of their own. This principle follows on to the above principle. No two groups are exactly alike due to the different parts or rather individuals that make up each group. An occupational therapist should not try to follow a specific generic programme where all groups are exposed to the same themes. Each group has their own identity and as such has their own specific needs. No group can be copied. Although highly unlikely, even if two groups were identically represented with the same diagnosis, gender, race and age together, the two groups will behave in different ways and have different dynamics. Each person brings his/her own background, experience, stereotyping, biases, likes and dislikes, thoughts, emotions and personality to the group. These aspects can never be matched. They slowly start by getting a feel for each other, by setting norms, and participating in activities. Yet some group members may not agree with the norms but keep quiet, comply or offer alternatives. The group members each have to decide how they will behave. By certain members complying and others being stronger, the group develops expectations and norms. Some issues are not easily resolved and the group members start to have two poles: for and against. However, for the group to function properly, the issue will need to be resolved at some stage. Once that specific issue has been resolved this new norm, contributes to the group's identity. As the group members find a way to work together and to adjust to the group, the group as a whole forms their own covert and overt group norms, causing the group's identity to develop. One group will allow group members to come to their group in slippers or with bare feet, but they have difficulty to resolve the issue of how much each person is expected to share. Another group battles to deal with an issue of 'realness' and resolves it by setting the norm of 'you can participate whenever you want to, but whatever you share needs to be real'. Each group will approach activities/ tasks differently. This makes group session exciting because each group is unique.

The practical implications are similar to the above; not pre-empting the group's choices or progress and allowing the group to deal with their specific issues in their own time and in their own manner. A solution or norm identified by one group will be rejected by another group. This emphasises the importance of allowing the group, as a whole, to make choices and to be accountable for their choices. Give observations and problems back to the group so that they can come up with their own solutions. An activity that facilitates the forming of a group's identity is to request the group to design their own group poster which must display a name, a logo and a motto appropriate for the group and what they wish to achieve within the time span of their group.

4.11   GROUP WISDOM

In psychodrama, there is a term Tele (Moreno 1946) which refers to the deep and profound wisdom that any group possesses as a collective. Group members connect with each other, both consciously and unconsciously, and because they participate and share experiences, the group develops wisdom about their group members and about the group process, that the occupational group therapist has difficulty accessing. Therefore, placing the responsibility of the groups' process on the group and giving the group opportunities to make their own decisions allow time for the group to tap into their own wisdom.

An example of this is as follows: In one group there were only a couple of minutes left and the occupational therapist requested the group to select a person in the group whom they wanted to hear more from. A couple of group members had brought their issues to the table varying from very superficial to deep topics. In the end the group elected to explore a superficial issue, much to the occupational therapist's surprise and concern. The decision was contrary to her/ his expectation of that specific group. The following day the occupational therapist asked the question and the group responded by explaining that they were emotionally tired and felt they would not do the deeper topic justice. The group wisdom is present in all groups and often leaves the group leader in awe. It is important that the occupational therapist allows the group to assert their wisdom and not to question the decision but rather ask for clarification and reflection on their decisions.

Occupational therapists that are still new to group therapy often try to steer the group process and should ask her/himself 'How much do I trust my group, to come to their own answers or make the decisions that are currently the correct one for the group? Do you trust that the group will do exactly what it needs to, when it needs to?' Often the answer is closely related to the follow-up question 'To what extent do you trust yourself with a group?' More experienced occupational therapists that have learnt to effectively facilitate or lead the group from behind have learnt to trust the group, and panic less. They know that sometimes groups need to enter uncomfortable places in order to resolve powerful issues. Groups in which the occupational therapist trusts his/her wisdom and process become incredibly effective in healing spaces.... it can even be described as sacred moments. These are moments in which occupational therapists become humble witnesses.

4.12   GROUP TECHNIQUES

There are specific group techniques that enable the occupational therapist to achieve the goal of improving mental health care user's social participation. These techniques are like a tool box which the therapist selects tools from to use at any given moment when a group is interacting and to facilitate further interactions and reflection. There is not always necessarily *one* correct technique to select as different techniques are appropriate but will lead to powerful discussion. One technique is not necessarily better than another.

4.12.1   Interaction

The group model described in this chapter is called the Interactive Occupational Therapy Group Model. The term 'interactive' is of essence and implies that interaction is imperative. Interaction can be defined as 'to have an effect on one another' or 'mutual or reciprocal action or influence'. This implies that group members need to provide opportunities to influence each other, to not just talk but to engage or connect. There must be a two-way process present for group members to have an effect on each other. Just saying something and then having the occupational therapist respond or ask the next question does NOT constitute interaction. Each person could just as well be seen individually. Group members need to be given the space and opportunity to react to anything happening inside the group.

The occupational therapist facilitates interaction by selecting activities where people need to connect with each other, physically or emotionally or to complete activities together. The warm-up activity of the carousel (see Chapter 9) is particularly helpful especially initially in groups, when the therapist is focused on building cohesiveness. In the carousel, two circles are formed, one within another where the group members face each other, one-on-one. The occupational therapist provides a topic to be discussed with a partner. The circle then moves on and a new partner is faced with a new topic to be discussed. The topics need not be deep but should provide opportunities to discover similarities or share topics that matter, for example 'one thing on your bucket list' or 'one dream you haven't dared to pursue'.

During group discussions, the group therapist should only pose questions occasionally and never make direct statements except the instructions for an activity and even then, she/he can end with, 'Is the group comfortable with that?' During a reflection, if nobody responds to a group participant, the occupational therapist can say for example, 'Who of you agreed with Mrs C? Tell us more about it?' Or 'Who differs in opinion? Explain to us'. Silence is also a powerful tool that can facilitate interaction as someone the group is bound to break the silence.

The OTIGM incorporates the term 'interactive' to ensure that group members are given an opportunity to play out their 'pathology' (for example voicing their prejudices, displaying their maladaptive matters) so that others can experience them and then provide accurate feedback about the impact this has on others, in the here-and-now. The interaction allows the group to form their own identity and to become greater than the sum of the individuals.

4.12.2   'I-Language' and Direct Communication

People often communicate their thoughts on a specific topic by making vague and ambiguous statements like: 'You tend to be in denial after losing someone'; or even more generalised 'People can often discuss sexual matters after a loss of a significant other'. Both these statements are vague and need to be dealt with as this type of communication leaves the conversation superficial. People may be affected by this and all respond by agreeing or disagreeing. When prompted to use 'I-language', the statement changes to 'I was in denial after losing my brother' or 'After losing my husband, I'm ashamed to say, I began to think of sexual matters'. The statement immediately becomes more emotionally charged, meaning people react more emotionally to the topic and to the person who made the statement. Fellow group members are either drawn to the person leading to a deeper connection or they can become more withdrawn. Group members may be evoked to respond on a deeper level than just agreeing or disagreeing on an intellectual level. If the group members engage with the topic on a deeper level, then the interaction takes on a different quality.

'I-language' causes group participants to take ownership of their engagement and responses. Initially the occupational therapist needs to actively facilitate 'I-language' by say pertinently '*It is necessary in this group to talk in the first person for example "I feel" or*

"I think" and avoid saying "people normally _____" or "one can expect _____" or even "we _____", since we cannot talk for others. We need to commit to what we are saying and it helps to say "I"". Other alternatives: 'You can't talk for other people, say I ...' or 'Restate what you just said by saying I feel ... or I am ...'. Some groups will make a joke of it or even exaggerate it in the first group or two, but the occupational therapist should not become discouraged and continue to actively encourage 'I-language'. After a while, it becomes a norm within the group and group members automatically start merging it into their conversations without noticing.

In combination with 'I-language', the occupational therapist needs to actively facilitate direct communication. Talking about someone does not have the necessary impact compared to talking TO the person involved. Compare for example if someone says *'Mrs X is a kind person'* on the one hand and if the same person looks Mrs X in the eye and says *'You are a kind person'*. The second example causes a more visceral response which again increases the quality of the engagement and leads to a deeper connection. During the first few groups, the group members need to develop the language necessary for direct communication. The group therapist should be patient as group members learn this way of communicating. Direct communication can be facilitated by the group therapist saying directly *'Tell him/her what you said and rather say You ...'.* For example the person may say *'I think Mrs G is not sharing sufficiently in this group'.* The therapist can intervene with *'Could you please repeat that by looking at Mrs G and saying to her I think you are ...'.* Mrs G is now given an opportunity to respond to this statement, once again looking and speaking directly to the person who made the statement. Once the group members get used to this way of talking, the therapist can later just point to the person involved and the group members will realise that it means they have to speak directly to the person. The group therapist can also avoid eye contact by subtly looking down when group members speak directly to her instead of to the group. The person talking will then look around the group and find someone else who is open to eye contact.

When a group is superficial, passive or stuck and moving around in circles, it indicates that the group members are starting to disengage. By facilitating in 'I-language' and direct communication, the group will immediately change the level of engagement of the group members.

4.12.3   Process Illumination

There are two aspects to the process illumination technique and both need to be present, otherwise the therapeutic power will not be effective. The first part could be summarised as the 'emotional' part where group members are made aware of their feelings and how their emotions change throughout the group towards different group members and during different activities. The group therefore is made aware of their experience in the here-and-now. The second part is the 'cognitive' part and named 'illumination' which so beautifully describes the process of standing outside the experience/group and trying to make sense of it. What could this reaction mean or where does this come from? The group then recognises, examines and tries to understand the group process. The group as a whole reflects on its own interactions and strives to integrate the experience.

The occupational therapist should be observing the group process/group dynamics which implies being aware of the group's interaction, the energy levels, the atmosphere or climate within the group. The group therapist can make comments like '*How are you feeling now after Mr H has shared his painful feelings with you?*' This would be to facilitate the experience: what exactly are the group members experiencing? Then the group therapist can facilitate the next step, i.e. illumination of the process immediately afterwards or he/she can keep it in mind and wait for a more appropriate moment either within the same or the next group. The facilitation can be something like '*I have noticed that every time a group member shares something painful with the group, the group members become restless or try to change the topic. What is happening with the group that we are observing this reaction? Who would like to try to explain this?*' The group therapist can also facilitate step two by saying '*I observe the group has suddenly become irritated. What is happening in this group at this moment?*' The group members may offer different viewpoints or experiences or explanations. It is not for the group therapist to draw a conclusion but to give it back to the group, allowing them the opportunity to make sense of their reactions.

This is an example of an incidence that occurred within a group to illustrate process of illumination: The group was waiting to start and group members were still arriving. A young man came into the group and said, he felt hurt because the group forgot his birthday. He made a big event of it and eventually after much prompting from him, the group members sang 'Happy Birthday' to him. Some group members shook hands and hugged him, congratulating him. The group hardly settled down when the young man burst out laughing saying he had fooled everyone; it was not really his birthday. Needless to say, this evoked strong feelings. The group therapist then asked the group members what they felt about this situation at that moment. Some said they were fine because nobody got hurt and the young man was just making a joke. Others were angry because at first, they did not believe him and from their experience described how they felt he 'forced' them to sing and now it proved they were right from the start. One young lady said it just proved to her that men could not be trusted. This was the first step, the experience. However, after this incident, the young man was overtly 'pushed out' of the group. Nobody wanted to partner him and the group members would interrupt him when he spoke or they would try to prove anything he said wrong. During a group later in the week, the occupational therapist asked the group members to observe how their reaction towards the young man changed since the group sang 'Happy Birthday' and asked the group to reflect on this. The group members gave the young man feedback about how his behaviour impacted on them. However, this is not sufficient for the process of illumination. The occupational therapist then asked what the reason was for the group to be 'convinced' by the young man when they instinctively knew he was untruthful. The reflective loop (otherwise known as illumination process) revealed that the group as a whole did not trust their own instincts which lead them to be easily convinced otherwise which left them feeling annoyed with themselves. The group examined issues of trust within the group as well as their ability to trust their own instincts. This example clearly illustrates the power and value of the process of illumination. The occupational therapist will at this stage ask the group members if they would like to participate in an activity that explores means of trusting the group members in this group in the here-and-now. If the group agrees, the occupational therapist presents an activity that allows group members to experience trust. An example of a trust activity could be to do a 'trust walk' (see Chapter 9). The occupational therapist will know what activity will be most appropriate for that particular group.

4.13 ACTIVITY SELECTION

One of the most powerful techniques available to occupational therapists using the OTIGM is the use of activities and an activity analysis to select appropriate activities. As group members will play out their 'pathology', the occupational therapist can effectively use participation in activities to elicit a true reflection of clients' social

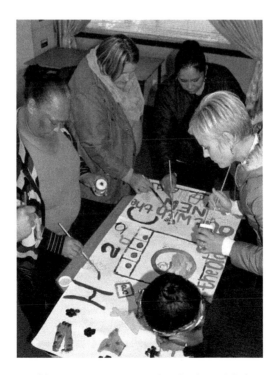

FIGURE 4.2 Making a group poster together (main activity).

participation and interpersonal relationships. In an activity that requires trust, clients will react to the activity and group members in a manner that is in line with their ability to trust people in the outside world. People can report that they have no problem trusting people, yet when participating in an activity requiring trust, a true reflection is displayed. This affords the occupational therapist the ability to facilitate the here-and-now concept. Through self-reflection of their thoughts and feelings in specific moments during the activity, the client comes to deeper realisations of themselves. Fellow group members can provide feedback and observations as well, all based on moments of activity participation. The occupational therapist can even challenge the client to try something new in the group, in the activity at that very moment.

For example, she/he may ask '*What do you need as this moment to trust Mrs C in this activity?*' The answer could be '*I need her reassurance*', which can then be given by Mrs C and the mental health care user is then challenged to try again. In a strongly cohesive group, the person will feel safe enough to take a risk and with the risk taking comes a new experience, a new behaviour that creates a new pathway. A new way of 'doing' has been experienced. Change is not made by knowledge, but by new experiences, new behaviour. This in turn makes it easier for the 'new' behaviour to be implemented outside the group.

Activities therefore become a corner stone of the OTIGM. Similarly, when group members have a need for a specific theme to be addressed, the occupational therapist selects an activity which enables the theme to be met during activity participation. No longer are there long discussions that take place about the theme identified, but rather about group members' participation and experience during the activity. As regards the example of trust, if the group members voice that they do not think they really trust each other, which is hampering the group's progress, the occupational therapist selects an activity through which they need to trust each other, for example selecting the 'blind walk' activity (see Chapter 9). If group members say they struggle to adapt to change, the occupational therapist selects an activity through which they experience change and are required to adapt to change, during the activity, here, now. Again during or after the activity, group members reflect on their experience. If some group members managed to cope better than others, their wisdom is shared with the group and group members can be encouraged to participate in the activity again, trying to implement the new wisdom.

Occupational therapists have an advantage, being able to accurately analyse activities that will enable the group members to reach the theme. Activities used in a group is not the same as using narrative therapy, which is often fraught with defence mechanisms, but a powerful tool to be therapeutically used in the here-and-now. Activities such as these are very powerful and occupational therapists are highly trained in the use of them.

4.14   GROUP PROCEDURES

Occupational therapists starting out, who are unfamiliar with OTIGM, are encouraged to make use of the group procedures below. As the occupational therapist becomes more experienced, these tend to serve as a guideline. The advantage of staying with these group procedures is that after a while the group can anticipate the procedures and it creates security for themselves. Even though these procedures are written down step-by-step, the occupational therapist should direct the group in such a manner that these steps flow into each other. Each aspect of the group procedure has been incorporating specific therapeutic advantages. These will be briefly explained. The therapist should not announce each step, for example 'Now we are going to introduce ourselves' and then 'and now we will make the rules . . .', etc. The occupational therapist knows the guidelines /steps and moves through them seamlessly.

4.14.1   Steps in the Group Process

4.14.1.1   Introduction

Introduction ensures that all group members know everybody else's name and something else which allows for connections to be made. Remember nobody can be expected to be comfortable sharing something about themselves, if they do not even know all the group members' names. Use a fun question, not only to relieve the tension but also to facilitate universality ('I also enjoy that') and cohesiveness ('we are all enjoying something and are sharing'). For example, *'Say your name and tell us what gives you a kick in life'* or *'Say your name and name something on your bucket list'*. The occupational therapist starts off and provides an example by introducing herself first and sharing something significant. Group members can be encouraged to come up with questions themselves.

4.14.1.2   Rules/Norms/Guidelines

Next, the group members need to set up rules/guidelines/norms for the duration that the group will be meeting. The occupational therapist can ask *'What norms would you like this group to have?'* It is important that the group members list their own norms. In exceptional cases the occupational therapist can make suggestions or name issues that they need to addressed. For example: *'What about confidentiality?'* or *'Do you wish to have a rule for punctuality?'*

Group members may come up with unusual rules, e.g. *'Anybody in the group is allowed to come in slippers'* or *'Anybody can bring something to drink with them to the group'*. Unless, the proposed rule will be obviously harmful, the occupational therapist should try to have an open mind and not impose any rules from her/his side. This is the first covert indication to the group that they need to take responsibility for their own group and that the occupational therapist is merely a facilitator. If she/he takes responsibility at this stage of the group, then it becomes difficult to get the group to take ownership and move forward. The group members will be passive. They may think that it seems that the occupational therapist will do the work. Another way to indicate to the group that it belongs to them is the language they use. Explain that the rules/norms are not cast in stone but can be changed by removing, modifying or even adding more norms as the need arises with the progression of the group.

4.14.1.3   Meet Group Members on Their Emotional Level

Next the occupational group therapist asks the group members how they are feeling. There are specific reasons for this step in the group procedures. They are:

(i) It gives the occupational therapist a good idea of what emotional level the group, as a whole, is functioning on and what can realistically be expected from the group members. So in a sense it is an emotional barometer for him/her.

(ii) Knowing where the group members function allows the occupational therapist to meet them on that level. If they are excited and happy, she/he can reflect their enthusiasm for the activities and if they are anxious, she/he can incorporate more structure.

(iii) It allows the group members to 'unburden' issues or conflict from outside the group. If a group member has had an argument with someone prior to the group, this will bother and preoccupy him/her throughout the entire session, making it difficult for them to focus on the group theme and other members. The occupational therapist therefore provides an opportunity for the group members to briefly vent their feelings, freeing up their mental space and energy for the group.

(iv) From an individual point of view, it enables the occupational therapist to monitor the progress regarding each mental health care user's mood and affect.

There are different ways to meet group members on their emotional level. The occupational therapist could just ask '*Where is everyone, emotionally today?*' or '*How are you feeling?*' Be careful that mental health care users do not answer with the words '*fine*', '*tired*', '*ok*' or '*cold*'. These are not emotions and can be a sign of resistance, or a way to avoid talking about their feelings. It is important that the occupational therapist asks each group participant present. It is easy for the quieter group members or those struggling to identify their feelings to say nothing. In order to steer the group towards a deeper level, group members learn to identify and verbalise their feelings. The here-and-now technique requires that clients become aware of their emotions and can describe the impact someone else's behaviour has on them.

4.14.1.4   Warm-Up/Icebreakers (See Chapter 1 of Section 2 in This Book)

Often when group therapists grow 'lazy', this is one of the first things they skip, because it takes some preparation. Icebreakers generate energy in a group which helps prepare the group members for the rest of the group to follow. When an icebreaker or warm-up (term used interchangeably in this chapter) is used, the flow of a group seems more effortless and the participation is more active.

In order to judge whether an icebreaker will be effective, the following criteria can be used during selection of an icebreaker to determine whether a warm-up is good or not.

(i) Facilitates cohesiveness (group members do it together or share something of themselves).

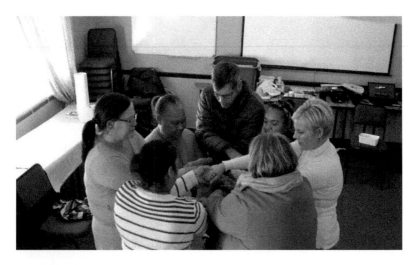

FIGURE 4.3   Warm-up. unknotting the human knot.

(ii) Facilitates interaction (they should talk directly to one another, NOT via the group therapist).

(iii) Decreases anxiety (there should be movement and group members should move out of their chairs).

(iv) Increases spontaneity (it should be fun and evoke laughter naturally).

(v) Introduces the theme of the group.

It may happen that some icebreakers do not meet all the criteria. For example if the theme selected is stress management, the group therapist may want the group members to experience some level of stress in order to introduce the theme; then it will not meet the criteria of decreasing anxiety. However the group therapist should aim to meet as many of the criteria as possible.

It is useful to measure icebreakers by counting the number of criteria met. For example a warm-up that only introduces the theme, is awarded 1/5 (20%). This is a poor warm-up. Likewise, a warm-up that meets four criteria is awarded 4/5 (80%) which is an effective warm-up. The author found from experience that using an effective

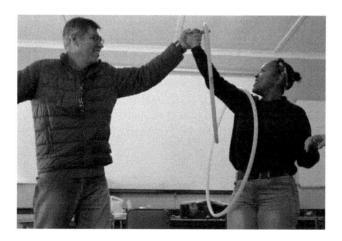

FIGURE 4.4   Sending the hula hoop around the group without letting go of each other's hands as warm-up.

warm-up results in a group 'half won'. Everything else flows so much easier from there, because the group members have energy and participate better.

4.14.1.5   Bridging

'Bridging' is a word that refers to the time period in the group that stretches from the end of the warm-up until the beginning of the activity; the group therapist leads the group members over the bridge which is not a jump, but a gentle, step-by-step guiding. There are basically three aspects that need to be incorporated during the bridging.

4.14.1.5.1   General Questions

The group therapist asks the group general questions concerning the warm-up and their experience of it. For example *'What was the warm-up like for you?'* or *'What did you experience during the warm-up?'* The group therapist can put observations made during the warm-up 'on the table' for the group members to respond to, e.g. *'Mrs X, I noticed you did not want to continue with the warm-up. Tell us about it'* or *'I noticed some of you chatted longer with specific group members than others. What prompted that?'* It is better to start off with a question directed to the whole group and then to focus on individuals. The aim of the general questions is to logically lead the group from introducing the theme in the warm-up to identifying the theme as something they would like to work on (problem spotting) and then to committing to the specific theme and activity for this group (contract).

4.14.1.5.2   Problem Spotting

During problem spotting, the occupational group therapist affords the group members the opportunity to identify a problem they have around the theme selected. If the group therapist has selected forgiveness as a theme, it would make no sense for mental health care users who are of the opinion that they do not need to forgive themselves or anyone else to be in the group; they would not give the necessary attention to the group. Problem spotting allows the group to consider the theme and gives them an opportunity to identify with it and 'buy into it'. Remember that the group therapist is facilitating a process. If the group feels they have no problem with the theme selected but identify a greater burning issue, e.g. trust, it is imperative that she/he follows the group process and changes her/his theme accordingly. After all, the group belongs to the group members and they need to take responsibility for the group process in order for the group to unfold. Problem spotting facilitates ownership of each group member. This also ensures that the group members are focused for the group and do not have to second-guess what the group is about. There are different ways to facilitate problem spotting. The easiest way to facilitate problem spotting is to ask members '*Do you find it difficult to …*'. Complete the sentence by incorporating the selected theme. For example: '*Do you find it difficult to think positively about yourself?*' (theme: increasing self-esteem) or '*Do you find it difficult to handle your stress?*' (theme: stress management). This question is posed to the group but each group member must answer it individually.

4.14.1.5.3 'Signing' a Contract or Committing to the Group/Activity

Once the group members have identified with the problem, it naturally follows that they are now open to commit to the activity and therefore to the rest of the group. If they have insight into the problem, they are more likely to commit and work towards addressing their problem. There are occasions when the group may not be ready and will therefore not commit. For example the group therapist may have selected a theme to explore taking less control and trying to 'go with the flow' within the group; yet at that specific time the group members may not be ready for it or feel there is another theme which takes priority. During the problem spotting question, they may all have agreed that they do find it difficult to just go with the flow, but when they need to commit or 'sign a contract', they are hesitant, maybe even resistant. Once again, remember that the group belongs to the group members and they should not be forced into an activity or process for which they are not yet ready. Therefore if they do not wish to commit to the theme selected, then the theme should be changed, at that very moment. The group therapist can then present these to the group members as alternatives or directly ask, '*If exploring going with the flow is not what the group would like to address today, what are other, more pressing issues are there at this moment?*' Alternatively she can ask the group '*I wonder what the reason is for the group not wanting to address issues of letting go of control?*'

The signing of the contract is more a verbal contract and is facilitated by means of a question: '*Would you like to …*'. The sentence is once again completed by incorporating the theme and activity. For example '*Would you like to take part in relaxation therapy in order to learn a method to handle your stress effectively?*' (theme: stress management). Or: '*Would you like to explore different ways to manage conflict?*' (theme: conflict management). Nobody should be coerced by the occupational group therapist into addressing their problems. This gives them the freedom and option to choose, but if they agree, it is as good as 'signing a contract' which they can be held accountable to. The group members need to 'sign a contract' individually and nobody can speak for anybody else in the group.

4.14.1.6   Activity

Once everyone has 'signed the contract' the group can proceed with the activity. The activity is *the* most important part of the group. It is through participating in the activity that the power of change lies. Occupational therapists are specialists in selecting appropriate activities after the necessary activity analysis has taken place. There are a few aspects to highlight with regard to the activity. Occupational therapists are encouraged to concentrate on selecting activities that create the here-and-now experience in direct relation to the group theme. This means that whatever the occupational therapist wants to address with the theme needs to be experienced within the group. If the theme selected is experiencing letting go of control and exploring going with the flow, an activity could be to paint with a partner's hand. The person holding the paint brush needs to have a balance between holding the paint brush firmly and at the same time, letting go control so that the partner can paint in any direction. If the group members merely draw or talk about the past situation or think about changing future behaviours, the group becomes a cognitive exercise with minimal opportunities to facilitate feedback, limiting curative factors like corrective emotional response and interpersonal learning. Little change can be facilitated when the focus is on the then-and-there. Groups that focus on past experiences will cause group members to disengage and the energy levels in the group decreases drastically. In order to select an activity that creates a here-and-now experience, the occupational therapist must be creative or innovative, yet the rewards are worth it. Instead of talking about adapting to change, develop an activity where group members need to constantly adapt to changes within the group. Observe their reactions. Remember the way group members reacted to change within this activity, here in this moment, is normally the way they react to change outside. The occupational therapist observes the group members' reactions and then facilitates reflection and feedback. If appropriate, the therapist can then challenge the mental health care user with new behaviour or new experiences, right now in the group session.

4.14.1.7   Post-Activity Discussion

By this stage the activity has been completed and now is the time to facilitate the post-activity discussion. In some groups, most of the therapy has already occurred and minimal reflection or discussion is necessary. The more effective the activity was in reaching the theme selected, the less post-activity discussion is required. However, it is good practice to ask group members what they experienced or to voice their experiences. It may be that the group members experienced a new insight or contrary experience, which will be a fruitful topic for the group to discuss. In the post-activity discussion, the occupational therapist facilitates, interaction, reflection and if appropriate feedback. For example a client may have made a sarcastic comment to another group member in the heat of the activity. The occupational group therapist can ask the person who was on the receiving end, what impact the comment made on them. She/he can facilitate self-awareness and ask the person who gave the comment what she/he was experiencing in that moment and what they hoped the comment would achieve. The group can now discuss more appropriate ways to deal with a similar situation.

A good way to get the post-activity discussion started is to ask the group members to describe to the group their experience of the activity. It is imperative that open-ended questions are asked in order to facilitate open discussion and interaction. Make sure that the group members talk in the first person and directly communicate with each other and not exclusively with the occupational therapist. Avoid asking specific group members questions, as it stifles the group and members are under the impression that they should only contribute or participate when they are addressed directly. Questioning should only be used as a last resort or if one group member avoids participation. Another option to facilitate interaction is to reflect back to the group observations made during the activity, for example *'Mrs Q, I noticed that is was more difficult for you to trust some group members than others. Tell us more about it'*. Alternatively, the group therapist can reflect on a specific mood or behaviour change in the group *'I notice that the energy levels in the group are very low right now, in contrast to during the activity. I wonder what the meaning of this is'*. Even process of illumination can be facilitated, e.g. *'Let's take a look at what has happened to the group's energy levels throughout the group. Who would like to venture an explanation?'* The occupational therapist can also facilitate feedback between group members: *'Mrs X I noticed the group did not respond to any suggestion you made? What was the impact of this on you?'* Remember, sometimes just asking a question can be therapeutic, as it compels group members to reflect more deeply and not all questions require a response.

The secret is for the occupational group therapist to limit all opinions or input from her/his side, even if she/he considers it to be therapeutic and to set a challenge for herself/himself, to ONLY ask questions and NOT make any comments or NOT to give any advice. Most groups will get to their own answers. Facilitate interaction by posing questions. When one person responds, use the response to 'keep the ball rolling'; for example, *'Who agrees with Mrs Q's view'* or

'Do you have another perspective/is your experience different?' Just posing a question to the group and then waiting in silence is another means of facilitation. It is almost certain that somebody will break the silence and set the interaction in motion.

It is important for the occupational therapist to end the group when she/he senses the group is drawing to a close. Premature closure can be as detrimental as continuing after the group has naturally wanted to end. Not all issues will necessarily be addressed in a particular group, which is not necessary. The group will discuss those issues most pressing to the group as individual. The occupational therapist should allow the group members to choose at all times and to read the group process. Additionally, the occupational therapist should not force 'fixing' problems or ensuring everybody feels good before ending the group. This shows that he/she is taking ownership of the group. The occupational group therapist can check in with the group members and ask them how they would like to end the group, if a sensitive issue has not reached a conclusion, but the group session's time has come to an end. Often the group members will surprise the occupational group therapist with their innovative ideas.

4.14.1.8   Closure

Once the discussion has come to a natural end, the group can be closed. The closure offers an opportunity for the group to have a definite end, with regard to the group experience. It makes use of quiet reflection, introspection and summarising. The occupational therapist provides a chance for the mental health care users to anchor any core ideas which the group members would like to take forward with them. It also allows the occupational therapist to evaluate the group, listening to what worked and what was effective for the group members and what may not have had the necessary impact that was hoped for.

Normally the occupational therapist asks the group members a question like *'What would you like to take with you from this group?'* or *'What was most significant for you from today's group?'* or *'What stood out for you from today's group?'* The question is open-ended so group members can comment on the theme, or on any curative factors, which they experienced or even something within the group process. The occupational therapist can even emphasise a curative factor by asking for example '*Who meant the most to you in this group?*' or '*If you could get to know someone better in the group, who would you like to invite for a cup of coffee?*' It is unnecessary for him/her to make any further comments at this stage. If the group finds it difficult to leave due to strong cohesion, he/she can dismiss the group and/or stand up and open the door, to indicate nonverbally that the group has ended.

A summary of the interactive occupational therapy group procedure is as follows:

1. Introductions.
2. Rules/norms/guidelines.
3. Meeting group members on their emotional level.
4. Warm-up/Icebreaker.
5. Bridging:
   a. General questions
   b. Problem spotting
   c. Contract/commitment
4. Activity.
5. Post-activity discussion.
6. Closure.

Timing of the group is important especially when there is limited time available within a group programme. As a rough guideline it would be wise to plan a group by dividing it up into thirds. Therefore in a 60 minute group, the first third is spent on the introduction until the end of the bridging – where group members have committed to the activity. The next 20 minutes or third is spent on the activity, as the activity is core to the therapeutic benefits of the OTIGM. The last third or 20 minutes is then spent on the post-activity discussion and closure. Remember this is a guideline to be used in planning, but the occupational therapist is merely a facilitator and is led by the group process.

4.14.1.8.1 Narratives of Past Groups

Below are a couple of examples of past group experiences when the OTIGM was implemented. It is hoped that this will enthuse the reader to the OTIGM and to see the powerful affect.

In a group made of group members with diverse religious beliefs, a young lady shared with the group that she felt so close to the group members, but she was greatly saddened by the fact that they did not share her beliefs. On further exploration, she voiced that she felt people cannot fully understand or connect with her unless they share her Christian belief. After a discussion, the group identified the need to connect more deeply with each other. The group therapist then incorporated an activity through which each group members connected nonverbally with every other group member. The young adult was profoundly touched by the experience, realising that there are no words, thoughts or beliefs required to be able to connect and experience being truly seen by others; to truly connect to others is powerfully healing. No amount of discussion would have brought about the healing if the young adult did not experience it. Her stereotypes and prejudices have been shifted, her interaction with others outside the group has subsequently changed and she has become more grounded in herself.

A thin, scrawny young male was present in a group which included a strong, masculine man. During a warm-up, the group needed to fit all the participants on a piece of newspaper on the floor. In that moment, the strong man said to the young man, 'We, men can do this. You stand on the other side and reach for my hand. We, men can hold up the women'. The strong man's confidence in the young man's ability boosted him and as the men were holding the women up, the young man's whole demeanour changed – he lifted his head, he grew taller, his shoulders dropped. This experience was the precursor to a meaningful discussion later in the group, between the two men choosing significant partners for intimate relationships.

The group represents mini-society and in one group there was a mother who had a fraught relationship with her teenage daughter. In the same group was a young lady who had a difficult relationship with her mother. During a post-activity discussion, the daughter shared her pain of what her mother had said to her. At that moment the mother spoke up and said she has often said things to her daughter that she knew would hurt her and that she deeply regretted it. She went on to explain her emotions in that situation and she apologised to the young lady on behalf of her mother. The young lady was deeply moved and they hugged each other, finding healing at being heard and understood. Returning home, the young lady had a new perspective on her mother, similarly the mother had a new perspective on her daughter.

In a game where each group member had to protect another group member, the one male group member, actually picked up a woman who was trying to protect him and used her as a shield, not allowing her the freedom of choice or movement to protect him. After the game, the group made observations overt and asked the man about the behaviour he displayed. He admitted that he had been alone for such a long time that he learnt to be totally independent and trusted nobody to look out for him. The group challenged the man to try the game again, and to try just in this game, in this group to take the first step in learning to trust again, to give a group member the chance to protect him. He selected a group member he felt he could trust and he was afforded the opportunity to try again. After the second attempt, he said it was scary for him, but he was surprised to notice that he was much less tired compared to the first attempt.

4.14.1.8.2 Last Thoughts

The OTIGM provides a group with the means to take ownership of their own group and therefore responsibility for their own healing. The biggest gift the occupational therapist can give the group is to trust them and the group process implicitly: to believe that what should happen for the greater good of the group will happen and conversely that whatever happens is for the greater good of the group. This allows him/her the freedom to be a true facilitator without having hidden agendas than need to be met. She/he facilitates cohesiveness so that the group members feel so secure in their own group that they start taking risks. The cohesiveness creates the safe space for uncomfortable but necessary discussions and questions to take place, those questions that change stereotyping, prejudices, bringing group members to new experiences. To facilitate groups is a precious and sacred privilege. Group members will share their most authentic selves and as Yalom (1975) states, groups are the most honest places as it is a place people can become free to express emotions, voice fears, apologise, try something new, admit mistakes and failings and connect with others. In short, they become more authentically themselves. In groups, people feel the healing value of true relationships and take the changes that occurred in the group back home. Is this not the most incredible place to be? To be called to be a witness for what is the worst and the best in us as human beings. It is good – very good.

4.14.2   Conclusion

The OTIGM is a powerful model that makes use of interaction and active participation in activities for group members to improve their social participation. Through participation in the activity, group members become who they are and display their thoughts and behaviour that usually negatively impacts on their interpersonal relationships. The occupational therapist then facilitates the here-and-now, through feedback from others, self-reflection, process illumination and through 'I-language' and direct communication techniques which leads group members to become aware of the impact they have on others. Within the group setting, they are now challenged to change one thought or action or behaviour within the group. A new behaviour creates a new pathway which in turn leads the way for healthier patterns or habits not only inside but also outside the group. The OTIGM uses occupational therapist's strengths of activity analysis and the use of activities to improve clients' social participation. By following specific group principles, using described techniques and tools, following the group procedures and participation in activities, occupational therapists will be amazed at the how effective the OTIGM can be. In a world where people are electronically connected but losing the skills of deep human connect, the role of occupational therapist will become increasingly important to help people reconnect through and with their humanness.

The reality is that people with disabilities are part of life: part of families, part of communities, part of society. This group was afforded the growth opportunity to converse and understand, on a deeper level, not only issues around disability but the lived experience of a person with a disability.

The value of this technique is that each individual can practise and become skilled in their social skills and form healthy relationships within a safe environment. People can experiment within the group because it represents society. After the group sessions, all the skills and insights learnt within a group are then easier to 'transfer' back to society, because the difference between a group and society is minimal. For example a person who finds it difficult to make eye contact, which is a requirement from society, can safely practise during groups until the skill is established. When the person is discharged, he will be able to make eye contact with ease, as he has been doing it with group members and it is a small step from the group members to community members.

It is very important to note that this concept is developed by the expertise of occupational therapists and the remarkable development in the profession, especially in occupational group therapy. All aspects of social skills and building interpersonal relationships can be addressed and practised in the group between group members. Once the skills have been mastered, the chances are good that long-term change has taken place and that building interpersonal relationships will no longer be a distant concept for each group member after they leave the group.

CHAPTER 5

Core Skills and Concepts

5.1 TRUST

Trust of the group leader, of other group members, the group process itself and of one's self is often lacking in the early stages of a group. The reasons for this can be complex but generally centres round the fear of failing or looking ridiculous. It can also centre round uncertainty as to what the group member will be expected to do or say or even expected to learn and possibly be rejected because of it. Sometimes memories of former unsatisfying learning experiences can get in the way. 'Fear and distrust are common behaviours in the early stages of groups, and as groups grow those fears gradually become less' (Bundey et al. 1984).

There is no doubt that a basic lack of trust amongst group members inhibits communication. If a group member feels that he/she may

Occupational Group Therapy, First Edition. Rosemary Crouch.
© 2021 John Wiley & Sons Ltd. Published 2021 by John Wiley & Sons Ltd.

get a negative response he/she is not likely to participate fully in the group. Trust develops in a group through openness, sharing, acceptance and support and cooperative intentions (Bundey et al. 1984). According to Fouché, activity in the introduction of the group and warm-up exercises at the start of the group helps develop the trust needed by the clients.

A group loses its spontaneity and therapeutic value if trust is lacking. It is therefore an essential element. It is not difficult to pick up a lack of trust in a group member. He/she will often show a hesitance to or avoidance in discussions about personal experiences and feelings, may sidetrack the group onto concrete tasks and subjects, be quite formal and be in a hurry to get the group finished.

5.2   DEFENCE MECHANISMS

If a group member feels threatened and fearful, and as already stated that if she/he does not trust the group, defence mechanisms will become evident. The client will defend him/herself by controlling or dissipating the anxiety. Common defence mechanisms, defined originally by Freud, to look out for are:

- 'Rationalisation where one constructs rational or acceptable reasons for actions of dubious merit.
- Repression – banishing unpalatable ideas, feelings, conflicts to the unconscious realm.
- Reaction formation in which one presents the opposite emotion or behaviour to what is really there, unconsciously (being over solicitous towards someone you hate).
- Displacement of an emotion provoked by one person/object on to a "safer" one (kicking the dog instead of the boss).
- Regression is functioning in a manner appropriate to an earlier stage of development (where responsibilities are less demanding).

- Projection – ascribing one's own unacceptable wishes and impulses to others.
- Intellectualisation – substituting intellectual processes for emotional ones, as a way of not dealing with the feelings already there' (Bundey et al. 1984).
- Denial – completely denying that a problem exists. This can be very deep seated.

5.3   TRANSFERENCE AND COUNTERTRANSFERENCE

Transference is the investment of emotion in the therapist/group leader (this applies to a therapist in any profession). The client may feel the love or hatred, dependence or rebellion, rivalry or rejection towards the group leader, that he has felt but never fully acknowledged for other people in his life – people whose impact has been earlier and inescapably close – people such as his parents, his first love, friends or enemies, heroes and villains of his childhood. It is considered to be a distortion of perception and the comparison may be inaccurate. It must be remembered that often transference can lead to dislikes and attractions that cannot be explained (Bundey et al. 1984).

Countertransference is where the occupational therapist may let emotions related to her/his previous encounter with people interfere with the relationship with the group member. Again this may be the angry child or a person most loved etc. It tends to foster favouritism and added attention but conversely can lead to the occupational therapist avoiding or not paying attention to the group member.

Moreno (1975) uses the word 'tele' to describe a good relationship with a client or group member which is a close rapport with the person which needs to exist if they are preparing to work together in psychodrama. It is not quite as strong as transference and countertransference. However the group leader needs to be very aware of transference, countertransference and tele as she/he must be aware of any factor influencing the group process.

5.4   GROUP FORMAT AND STRUCTURE: STAGES AND PHASES OF GROUP DEVELOPMENT

In a modern climate it is the responsibility of the occupational therapist to select the clients for the group according to the assessment that has taken place which is absolutely vital to the whole process. Referrals from other professionals must be screened and assessed before the person is placed in a group. There must be good structuring of the group according to personalities, levels of functioning and the medical/psychiatric illness. From experience the author warns against homogeneous groups such as a group of middle-aged depressed women or a group of adolescents all with conduct disorders and attention deficit hyperactive disorder (ADHD). Heterogeneity brings in different interests and controlled liveliness and is highly recommended.

The The Vona du Toit Model of Creative Ability [VdTMoCA] (2019) and the activity participation outcome measure (APOM) (Casteleijn 2014) are very appropriate assessments for the occupational therapist to use in order to determine the functioning level of clients before allocating them to a group. The venue is very important for the success of the group therapy and must include an interruption-free environment. The size of the group is very important and 8–12 group members seem a good estimate in order to carry out effective therapy. Large groups of 15–20 clients are ineffectual even if they are involved in creative activities. It is not recommended. Where group members are severely disabled as in an acute setting, the smaller the group should be with four being the lowest count.

The actual physical structuring of a group is extremely important. Never have the group leader facing a row of clients – this set up fosters confrontation! A well-spaced round group where all group members have a clear view of each other, whether he/she is sitting on a chair or the floor, is recommended.

Groups with young people and adolescents tend to be much more relaxed and this should be encouraged. The group leader and co-leader should not sit together.

A basic suggestion of the format of occupational group therapy is as follows:

- The group leader and co-leader introduce themselves.
- There must be an explanation of the purpose of the group and is necessary for the setting of goals. Introduction of the subject of the group takes place.
- The group members greet each other and new members introduce themselves.
- Confidentiality must be stressed.
- Then there is the warm-up phrase and warm-ups and ice-breakers are described in Chapter 8.
- The interaction takes place.
- The occupational group therapists must undertake a periodic recap of goals and possible conflict resolution.
- The next step is the summary including the goals achieved, conflicts resolved, sometimes and a discussion on individual participation, roles taken up and future plans.
- The closure is extremely important and includes the reminder of confidentiality and a final comment, without falling into the trap of reopening the subject.
- Thanks and termination must take place automatically.
- In the case of psychodrama and other intense groups, a safe environment is provided where clients can discuss their vulnerability. It is called the recovery room.

To summarise the above discussion by combining the thoughts of various theorists one could say that the phases of group development are as follows:

- Phase I: Forming – establishment of a common base
- Phase II: Storming – time of conflict
- Phase III: Norming – resolution of conflict
- Phase IV: Performing – consensus and maximum productivity (Tuckman 1981).

5.5   CULTURAL INFLUENCES IN OCCUPATIONAL GROUP THERAPY

When addressing the profession of occupational therapy, Gujral states that 'Cultural factors have potentially far-reaching effects on the provision of care, including selection and interpretation of assessment instruments, interpersonal communication, and intervention and outcome expectations' (p. 472 Gujral in Creek 2002). Guijral also states that 'Models for the practice of occupational therapy, such as the model of human occupational (Kielhofner), urge us to include culture as an integral component of the clinical reasoning process, as we consider complex interactions between the individual and the environment' (p. 483).

Unless one is working in a particular rural or urban environment with the local community, it is likely that the occupational group therapist will have people of different cultures in the group. 'Culture has long been defined with respect to its underlying influence on individual views, or in terms of its artistic or scientific expression. It is, however, unfortunate that culture in today's society is often immediately replaced with the idea of race or ethnicity, as well as the prejudgements that may accompany those ideas. It is important to note that neither race nor ethnicity is synonymous with culture' (Townsend and Polatajko 2007, p. 52).

It is partly because of the fact that occupational therapists use interactive techniques that can include close contact with another group member, that cognisance must be taken as to the culture of group members. For example a religious Jewish or Muslim man may not touch a woman in the group, particularly if the group members are holding hands. In some African cultures a woman may not look straight into a man's eye as it seen as a sign of disrespect and a man who looks directly into the eyes of another man may appear to be aggressive. This is particularly important when addressing assertive behaviour. It may also not be a cultural norm to talk about one's family members in a group or interact with them as in psychodrama. 'The approach to cross-cultural work must be that of open-mindedness, acceptance and positive attitude towards different cultures' (Voce and Ramukumba in Crouch and Alers 1997, p. 127).

It is true to say that there is a very big diversity in psychosocial issues when working as an occupational group therapist and each culture is unique. It is therefore imperative that she/he is fully aware of the cultural background of each group member which can be determined during the assessment. It also may come to light in the first stages of group work and is often associated with religious beliefs. Unless the group is a specific religious group, it is not wise to get onto the subject of religion as it often causes tension. However, it is important that individual group members acknowledge and respect the culture and religion of others and often this has to be dealt with when the group is in the 'forming' stage.

The words of Annah Lesunyane sum up this section by saying 'the use of activity as therapy is very powerful and relates directly to that which is identified to be within that social and cultural context' (Lesunyane 2010 p. 56 in Alers and Crouch).

CHAPTER 6

Clinical Reasoning, Clinical Thinking and Ethical Reasoning Relating to Occupational Group Therapy

6.1 CLINICAL REASONING AND GROUP WORK

> Vision without action is only a dream,
> Action without vision just passes the time,
> Action with vision can change the world.
> (Joel Arthur Barker 1991)

What is clinical reasoning? It is a way of thinking, a cognitive process whereby the occupational therapists can better understand clients

Occupational Group Therapy, First Edition. Rosemary Crouch.
© 2021 John Wiley & Sons Ltd. Published 2021 by John Wiley & Sons Ltd.

and their problems and draw conclusions whilst they are undertaking routine occupations (Reed and Sanderson 1983).

Well-known theorists in occupational therapy such as Townsend (1999), Alers and Smuts (2002), Sinclair (2003) and Creek and Bullock (2008) have written extensively on this subject. There is no intention of repeating their work here because it is easily accessible, but the tie up with group work must be discussed. Included, however, are some of Vivyan Alers' wise words which pertain to occupational group therapy.

Clinical reasoning is intimately involved with critical thinking. In occupational group therapy, it is often just the smallest change in a client's social behaviour that makes the most impression. 'These individual gems of improvement need to be remembered and the "reflection on action with vision" needs to be considered. This is how occupational therapists can develop their clinical reasoning powers to progress from a novice to an expert' (Alers in Crouch and Alers 2014, p. 67).

'Clinical reasoning is a complex procedure incorporating personal knowledge, theoretical background and an application of cognitive abilities to integrate information for treatment intervention. This process is greatly enhanced by clinical and life experience. Clinical reasoning is the "what?", "how?" and "why?" for "best practice" in occupational therapy. These questions are all interchangeable for the "best practice" model to emerge from the clinical reasoning. Clinical reasoning also involves the processing of constantly changing data and circumstances. Critical thinking is the foundation for this process to happen. The "best practice model" has developed from therapist directed to client-centred, family-centred or community centred practice. This relates to the challenges of where the role of control lies' (Robertson 2012).

The elements of critical thinking are the generic starting point for clinical reasoning. The eight-step critical thinking process leads the person to factual evidence to be able to proceed to the clinical reasoning process (Paul 1996) as follows:

1. Purpose – this is the goal which needs to be realistic and achievable. The range of the purpose can be significant to trivial and it needs to be consistent and not be contradictory.

2. Question at issue – this is the problem to be solved. The importance of the problem needs to be considered as well as the requirements for solving the problem.

3. Assumptions – these are the things taken for granted. When looking at assumptions they need to be recognised and articulated clearly and considered whether they are justifiable or not, crucial or extraneous, consistent or contradictory.

4. Implications – further implications and consequences will always arise no matter where the reasoning is ended. It is necessary to identify whether the implications are significant and realistic.

5. Inferences – these are the steps of reasoning. This refers to the logical progression of 'since this happens, that will also occur'.

6. Point of view – this is a frame of reference. The point of view is aimed at being broad, flexible, fair and adhered to consistently.

7. Concepts - this is the conceptual dimension of reasoning, including theories, principles, axioms and rules implicit in the reasoning.

8. Evidence – this is the empirical dimension of reasoning, namely the experiences, data or raw material. This needs to be reported clearly, fairly and accurately (Figure 6.1).

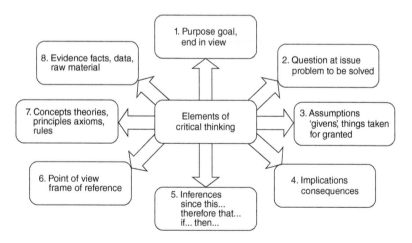

FIGURE 6.1   The eight sequential stages of critical thinking. *Source:* Crouch and Alers (2014).

'So often occupational therapists have too high expectations for the improvement of their patients/clients (relating to their own value systems instead of having a client-centred approach and the accompanying client's value system), thus not realistically evaluating their intervention outcomes' (Alers in Crouch and Alers 2014, p. 68).

Reflective judgement indicates the personal ability to weigh arguments and make 'best' decisions. Epistemological beliefs lay the foundation for judgement in all situations, including clinical encounters. Understanding one's own beliefs and biases is fundamental in developing into an expert reflective practitioner (Sinclair 2003 in Crouch and Alers p. 75).

Clinical reasoning is a term described by Unsworth in 2016 as the thinking processes of therapists when undertaking clinical practice and she also describes it as practice decision making. This is a simplistic but succinct way of describing the concept.

Jennifer Creek in Alers and Crouch (2010) states that 'At each stage during an intervention, the occupational therapist has to think carefully, evaluate the situation and decide on the most appropriate course of action' (p. 112). This is borne out by Fouché (see Chapter 4) and is relevant to the occupational therapists' personal and practice contexts when carrying out group work. Scholl and Cervero (1993) state that 'Examples of therapists' contexts are a repertoire of therapy skills, ability to read the practice culture, negotiation skills and personal motivation' (p. 609).

The relevance of this concept to occupational group therapy lies in the fact that it incorporates the cognitive process and way of thinking that therapists use to understand clients and make conclusions on the basis of the information that is available (Reed and Sanderson 1983; Hagedorn 2000). It is much the same in all therapy as it encourages the good use of theory, develops best practice and particularly in group work ensures safety of practice.

In the author's opinion interactive reasoning, such as collaborative reasoning, as described by Hagedom in 2000 is most frequently used in group work. This type of reasoning constructs a shared language of actions and meaning to determine whether the group is going well. It also has to do with ethical and moral reasoning (Perimal 28 September 2014 SUNIRTAR web). (See the next section on ethics.)

6.2   ETHICAL REASONING: CONSIDERATIONS IN LEADING A THERAPEUTIC GROUP

There are certain ethical considerations that need to be addressed when considering group leadership in occupational therapy. The area of ethics is sometimes overlooked and yet is an important starting point for examining responsibilities and values:

- Keep and protect the confidentiality of group members by clearly defining what it means and why it is important and the risks and difficulties involved in the enforcement. This should take place at the commencement of every group meeting.
- Explain the risks and difficulties that may occur when involved in participating in the group. This why confidentiality is so important and why group members can learn to trust each other.
- Respect and encourage the voluntary participation of group members so as to promote their independent participation.
- Refrain from developing intimate personal relationships with group members throughout the duration of any group programme.
- No recording or secret observation of group sessions may take place without the permission of group members/parents (e.g. in the case of children).
- Do not allow group members to impose their personal agendas and values on group members.
- Do not use any technique or intervention unless thoroughly trained in its use.
- Provide information to group members about any special technique or activities in which they are expected to participate.
- Respect the religious, cultural views and norms of group members.
- There must be no sexual discrimination of any kind (Van der Reyden and Crouch 2014).

Van der Reyden and Crouch in 2014 also defined the universally accepted principles of patient care in any circumstances as:

- Considering the needs of the patient/client above all else (beneficence).
- Doing no harm (non-maleficence).
- Respecting autonomy and providing equitable services (justice).

These principles underpin all conduct and Practitioner–patient/ client relationships.

CHAPTER 7

Styles of Group Leadership and Co-leadership: Guidelines to Address the Differences Including Working with Other Professionals

7.1 GROUP LEADERSHIP

There have been various attempts to define styles of group leadership by the well-known group theorists such as Carl Rogers, Joseph Moreno and Linda Findley. By experience one understands that professionals have styles that develop over time and are related to the profession in which they find themselves. In Bundey et al. (1984) stated that 'No style of leadership is right or wrong. Depending on the personality of the leader, the goals of group members, their

Occupational Group Therapy, First Edition. Rosemary Crouch.

present level of functioning and the purpose of the group, effective leadership may involve quite different behaviours on the part of the leader' (p. B15). The group leader does have a strong influence on the group which directly affects group functioning. A client-centred approach, as stated by Fouché in Chapter 4, is extremely effective and in strongly therapeutic group work the needs and feelings of the group members are uppermost. The structure of the group is important as is the attainment of goals.

There are three broad categories of styles of group leadership described by Bundey et al. (1984). These are:

1. Autocratic leadership: Autocratic leadership is directive in nature and the leader maintains the leadership role at all times. This would only be suitable (if at all) when chairing a meeting where the leader determines what has to be done and is very focussed on the task at hand. In this case the group members are not involved in the decision-making process.

2. Democratic leadership: In occupational group therapy, the qualities of effective group leadership are democratic; they consult with group members and involve them in the decision-making process. They may share the leadership role and the tasks of the group leader. They consider both the task of the group and the maintenance of membership as important. They should have meaning attribution, be caring, and have effective communication and self-awareness. A democratic group leader should nevertheless have executive functioning and be in control of the group at all times, even 'leading from behind' as discussed by Fouché in Chapter 4.

3. Laissez-faire leadership: This type of leadership was employed by psychotherapists such as Carl Rogers. It is a nondirective (may even be inactive) type of group leadership where the leader is very willing to share the leadership role and lets the group decide how things will be done. Amazingly enough the leader is very focussed on the maintenance of the group! The basic scope of the profession of occupational

therapy does not, in most countries, include psychotherapy; yet, taking a leaf out of the psychotherapist's book is sometimes appropriate particularly when working with high-functioning adults.

7.2   CO-GROUP LEADERSHIP

Working with co-leaders or being a co-leader of a group needs special consideration. Firstly, it is a privilege to work with other professionals in the field and it is an enhanced benefit to the clients but only if the leaders are similarly trained and have prepared well for the group.

In 2012, Kivlinghan stated that 'When it comes to group format, new research shows that two leaders are better than one. Members of co-led groups experience greater benefits than those of individually led groups. That second set of eyes and ears makes a big difference when group leaders are trying to follow multiple interactions'.

Sally Barlow (in Kivlinghan 2012) states that 'An individual group therapist, no matter how skilled, cannot keep up with the richness of the group experience'.

It must also be realised that co-leadership is a superb way to train other professionals or occupational therapists in group work. It is always a huge privilege to work with an experienced group leader. It is recommended that there only ever be one or two leaders of any group.

Bundey et al. (1984) describe two types of co-leadership, equal and unequal leadership. Equal leadership is where the two leaders have been similarly trained and have similar experience and unequal co-leadership which is usually used in training circumstances or where the co-leader is inexperienced. It is clearly stated that whatever the type of co-leadership is employed there must be thorough preparation beforehand; otherwise, the leaders will have a negative effect on the group. All aspects of the group must be discussed before the group starts. Some groups may tolerate disagreement of the two leaders but the majority will not. It will add to the group members' own confusion.

Processing of the group by the two leaders must take place afterwards. It is essential that any conflicts be resolved and that planning takes place for any further group work together.

7.3   WORKING WITH OTHER PROFESSIONALS IN GROUP WORK

In transdisciplinary and multidisciplinary teams, occupational therapists often have the opportunity to work with other professionals in group work. This may be as a leader, co-leader as already discussed, or just as a member of the team. In well-functioning teams, even if the professionals are differently trained, one professional can learn from the other. Areas of differences and friction should be ironed out. Openness and professional development should take place; otherwise, intervention will be compromised. Lloyd and Maas (1997) stated that 'the success of a group depends to a large extent on the skills, ability and attitude of the therapist. It is necessary to have a sound theoretical basis for group therapy, and to utilise a particular frame of reference depending on the orientation of the therapist'.

CHAPTER 8

Transdisciplinary Service Delivery

8.1 TRANSDISCIPLINARY SERVICE DELIVERY

In a number of sub-Saharan countries and countries globally where there is overwhelming poverty and resources are poor in the communities, the transdisciplinary service delivery is appropriate. It is very important for occupational therapists to look at therapeutic group work in this light and under these circumstances.

In Uys and Samuels (2010) described the transdisciplinary service delivery as follows: 'Within this model various professional disciplines work together at all levels, and roles are often blended to enhance communication. Family members are also active participants rather than passive recipients of information and intervention. Trans-disciplinary teams differ from the more traditional multidisciplinary teams in that team members commit to teach, learn and work across disciplinary boundaries in order to provide integrated services' (p. 220).

Looking at our previous chapters on the relevance of different models of intervention and in the discussion on core concepts and skills in occupational group therapy, one wonders how the transdisciplinary model works.

A sense of responsibility for the future of humanity along with trans-disciplinary action is crucial This may be our only defence. If we do not take up the challenges we will all be accomplices in creating and maintaining a sick society

(Max-Neef 1991).

It stands to good reason that group work is the obvious choice of intervention in under-resourced communities and the type of group work will be dictated by the position and training of the group leader. It is important to note, as in Crouch (2008), mid-level health workers (Community Rehabilitation Workers – CRWs) were successfully training in leading stress management groups in an impoverished society. Good group leaders can be trained.

Fouché (2020) points out that there is a difference in the use of groups which have a tangible outcome such as community planning groups, activity and open groups and smaller, emotionally charged therapy groups as described in the OTIGM (See Chapter 4). In the transdisciplinary scenario, there is a group leader and in the OTIGM there must be a highly trained therapist. Please refer to Section 1.2 where reference is made to the classification of group therapy and the level of emotional intensity.

However, whether it is group work or group therapy, the same power of using groups is relevant. The same dynamics, basic concepts and curative factors as defined by Yalom (1985) apply. Whether it is the occupational therapist, the physiotherapist, the speech therapist, the social worker, the family member or teacher who is the group leader, the same rules and ethics of group leadership apply (see Chapter 7 on styles of group leadership).

Another important factor in transdisciplinary group work is the client-centred approach (Law et al. 1994) which brings about empowerment to the community in which the team members work.

The decisions made are not those of the group leader but those of the community members. One must remember once again that the group leader does not make the decisions, the group members do! 'Empowerment at a community level is related to growth and development through shared vision and common goals and therefore families are important agents to bring about empowerment at a community level' (Uys and Samuels 2010, p. 209).

The other important factor is the 'grey areas' that exist between the professionals that work in a transdisciplinary team in the community, including teachers. When one looks at the variation in tasks in community work such as groups, individual and group counselling, working with politicians, finances, community leaders etc. it is obvious that professionals have to be flexible, use their common sense as well as use their own set of skills. The scope of the professions tends to become blurred. This could be a positive factor but from an ethical point of view a health professional may still not carry out an intervention for which he/she is not trained. This is particularly true of group work. It has been made clear in the previous chapters that a group leader must know (or have some guidance) how to lead a group or the consequences could be negative. When community members are leading a group, it is highly recommended that there is one professional co-leader especially when important decisions have to be made (see Chapter 7 on co-leadership).

THE PRACTICAL APPROACH TO OCCUPATIONAL GROUP THERAPY

CHAPTER 9

Warm-Up and Icebreaker Techniques

One of the distinguishing features of occupational group therapy has always been 'activity'. Vivyan Alers and the author, who worked together for many years, promoted this very important, vital aspect of group work not only in terms of having an activity as part of the group, but also in the style of group leadership. Moreno (1953) in his original work stressed the 'theory of spontaneity' which is fostered by the group leader being physically and cognitively active in the leading of a group as opposed to just sitting and talking. Carrying out warm-up techniques or icebreakers is a good example of this concept. Rosemary and Vivyan's training in psychodrama internationally fostered this ability to be active, and has become a very important part of occupational group therapy.

Usually warm-up techniques are used at the beginning of a psychodrama group or any other type of group but can also be used on its own as a group in itself. There are excellent authors in the profession such as Remocker and Storch (original publication 1977)

Occupational Group Therapy, First Edition. Rosemary Crouch.
© 2021 John Wiley & Sons Ltd. Published 2021 by John Wiley & Sons Ltd.

who developed their skills and published brilliant publications in this respect. Although the concept was not new the authors spoke out in their handbook (Action Speaks Louder) and published excellent, well-tried techniques as a practical handbook for occupational therapists. These include:

9.1   INTRODUCTION TO EACH OTHER IN THE GROUP

When the group members are well settled in positions where they can clearly see each other, either sitting or standing, and the group therapist is present, there needs to be an introduction. Here are a couple of examples:

- If sitting, one group member turns to the other next to him/her and says 'Hi I am (Joan, John etc. depending what they call themselves. Sometimes it can be Mrs Jones!) I am _____' They can shake hands if appropriate. The partner replies in the same way. This continues on around the group until everyone has introduced themselves. If preferred, the group therapist can ask group members to express a feeling such as 'I'm Joan and I am feeling very anxious'.
- If standing, one member of the group steps into the group alone and says she makes a physical movement like a bow or a wave. The other group members then step into the group and mimic what the group member has done and said. This really breaks the ice and it such fun. In one instance when working with students, a group member stepped into the group and said 'Hi I am Tina' and promptly did a perfect cartwheel to the surprise of the group members, who of course could not replicate the movement but had a good laugh.

9.2   THE CAROUSEL

This is versatile warm-up requiring some creative application by the occupational group therapist.

Group members sit on cushions on the floor in a group (chairs can be used if necessary). There is an inner and an outer group with the inner group members facing a partner in the outer group. An interaction between the partners is encouraged by the group therapist. This is often an introduction to each other for the first interaction 'I am Mary Jones, and I _____. Who are you?' After about five minutes the outer group moves one person to the right and then members are facing a new partner. The next exercise could be 'tell the person opposite something important that happened to you when you were a child (or a teenager etc.)'. This requires about seven minutes. The inner group then moves one person to the right, and so it goes until everyone has met everyone from the other group. (This means that each member has only met half of the whole group.) Have a short discussion after each exercise. Recommended exercises are :

- Stare into the eyes of the person opposite you without saying anything for a few minutes until told to stop. (Known as eye-balling and some people feel very uncomfortable especially some cultures. This is a good topic for discussion and group therapy.)
- Discuss a very happy incident in your life with your partner opposite.
- The people on the inner circle say 'yes you will' and the outer person says 'no I won't'. Do not say anything else; only these words. (Be warned that people tend to shout!)
- Sit back-to-back with your partner and see who can push the other one over. Discuss whether you are or are not a 'push over'.
- Sit quietly holding the hands of the person opposite to determine their strengths. Discuss with the partner only and then the group. The group leader uses her/his own ingenuity to develop appropriate exercises depending on the level of the group. Continue until half the group has met half the group and the last exercise can be just sitting quietly with eyes closed to calm down and bring closure. A brilliant discussion can then ensue and in psychodrama the protagonist is often identified in this process.

9.3　STICKERS

Each group member is given five sticky labels and a dark pen. They are asked to write a feature of themselves on each sticker and stick them on any part of their body so they can be seen. They then circulate in the group introducing themselves to everyone, e.g. 'Hi I am George and I am "jovial" and "serious at times" etc. This is a very popular technique and fun.

9.4　THE MAGIC SHOP

This is a great favourite in groups. The group leader asks the group members to imagine a small shop and they can set up a small table and chairs. Group members are asked to imagine all sorts of wonderful qualities on the shelves of this shop. Either the psychodramatist, a trained professional or a group member can be asked to be the shopkeeper. Members of the group go to buy concepts such as 'self-esteem' or 'confidence' and may also ask for 'good health'. At first it will be found that members are quite basic, e.g. they want to buy 'love' or 'happiness'. The shopkeeper can be quite creative asking simple questions and bargaining as to the cost. Blatner (1973) uses the example 'You want love from everybody? Well that will cost quite a bit more' (p. 41). Bargaining can also take place between shopkeeper and client and the client can consult with the members of the group. It can all be such fun but also very therapeutic. As Blatner says 'the magic shop is an excellent technique, not only for warming-up a group but also for the purposes of clarifying goals and examining the consequences of ones choices' (p. 42).

9.5　THE MAGIC BUS

This is a similar technique to the magic shop but this time there is a bus driver (the group leader or competent person) and about four to six chairs configured like a bus. Group members take up positions in the bus and tell the bus driver where they are 'going'. Again it is a concept such as 'I am going to a place called sobriety' or 'Would you please take me to inner peace'. The concept is taken up by the group, directed by the leader. Another group member may ask to go with that person on the bus.

9.6   THE MAGIC CARPET

The magic carpet is used frequently by Louise Fouché (see Chapter 4). The same concept applies as in the two warm-ups above.

A small carpet or big piece of paper is placed on the floor in the middle of the group. This is the magic carpet and it can go anywhere one desires. Group members go and stand on the carpet and declare to the group 'where they are going'. If others are going to the same place they climb on board too until the carpet is ready to go. A discussion ensues and sharing takes place. Once again the protagonist often comes forward in this type of warm-up and the psychodrama commences.

9.7   GUIDED FANTASY

Often this technique is preceded by relaxation and is not suitable for any group member who has a psychotic disorder or is not in touch with reality.

While in a relaxed state group members are asked to visit a place of fantasy in their minds such as a beautiful beach, a forest, a lovely garden, walking up a mountain and being in a special house. Suggestions can be made by the group members themselves but the guiding must be done by the group leader. The discussion afterwards is always very valuable.

It is also possible for the group to share a fantasy and this has been discussed by Leuner (1969).

9.8   SHARED DRAWINGS – 'ME, MYSELF AND ANOTHER ME' (AVNON 1989)

It is a wonderful priviledge for an occupational group therapist to work with a famous group expert and a good example of an expert in psychodrama is Esty Avnon from Israel, one of the leading psychodramatists in the world. The warm-up techniques that she uses are very creative, comfortable and extremely effective. 'Me, myself and another me' is a drawing technique where the group member interviews the two images that he/she has drawn/painted of the left and right character of him/herself. Esty worked in a spacious room and each group member had two pieces of A2 paper which was stuck onto the wall. A variety of drawing and painting materials were on hand and group members could choose their medium. One page was to represent the right character of themselves and the other piece of paper the left character. Each group member presented their pictures to the whole group and Esty led the discussion. The group member was asked to start a confrontation between the two sides of themselves represented in their pictures. Examples of the questions that one side asked the other were:

- Who are you?
- How old are you?
- What is your name?
- What do you look like?
- How do you feel at this moment?
- What do you think? And what would you like to say to me?
- What do **you** have to say to the other character?

Esty often intervened at the end and asked the group member to share the physical relationship between the characters, e.g. the posture and the way they face one another. She asked what the type of interpersonal relationship was between the two sides (familial or other) and what the nature of the relationship is between the characters (close, opposing, etc.). Other questions were 'where do you come from and what do you plan to do in the future?'

This is a delightful technique and highly recommended.

9.9   USING THERAPEUTIC ABSTRACT CARDS

Abstract cards were developed by Avnon (1989) and was followed by Alers (2007) who, as a typical occupational therapist, made her own cards. These cards are the same size as a pack of ordinary playing cards but have abstract or slightly more definable objects on each one. Esty developed various packs of cards, i.e. 'ecco cards' depicting abstract paintings, 'habitat' cards depicting the earth's natural environment, 'sailing into the world of magic' therapeutic storytelling cards depicting stories from cultural backgrounds and 'persona cards' portraits of a wide range of people. These cards are very easy to use. The occupational group therapist places a particular pack of cards on the floor or a table in the middle of the group spreading them out face up. She/he gives the group time to choose a card that resembles them or has some meaning for them. Each group member introduces themselves to the group using the card. Very often group members become involved at an emotional level and if using the technique of psychodrama the protagonist can easily be determined (Figure 9.1).

However, from experience these cards/or your own ones can be used to great effect in any group as a warm-up.

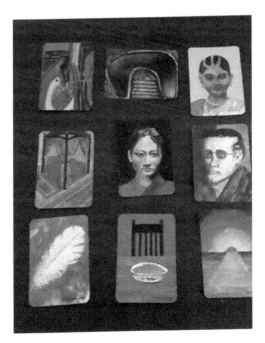

FIGURE 9.1 Examples of Esty's cards. *Source*: OH cards, used by Dr. Ofra Ayalon ect.

9.10   SCULPTING

This is a very powerful warm-up which is borrowed from the family therapy techniques but has been used for a long time by occupational group therapists in their groups. It is used as a group warm-up and is very popular with the group members because it gives them insight into the relationships with their families and others. According to Fouché (2020) this can easily become a group therapy interaction.

A group member who must offer to participate, or be very gently persuaded, is asked to choose family members from the group and place them in an emotional distance from him/herself. Each family member must be described and placed so that he/she faces the group member, is turned away, may be standing or sitting (or standing on a chair) and may possibly have outstretched arms towards him/her etc. If there are not enough group members chairs can be used instead. When everyone is in place the group members are asked about the way they feel about the placements and about their feelings standing in the middle of this family. Individual relationships can be discussed too. The group takes part.

This is a popular technique and often group members who are reluctant to participate in the group find this a good way to get involved. Often, again a protagonist for psychodrama can be identified.

9.11   THE EMPTY CHAIR (AUXILIARY CHAIR)

This is a major psychodrama technique which can be used both as a warm-up or as part of the psychodrama. The use in psychodrama will be described later.

It is important to note that a good level of cohesiveness must exist in the group before using this technique, group members must trust each other.

An empty chair is placed in the middle of the group. Group members are asked if they can visualise someone sitting in that chair. It could be just anyone or could be someone with whom they have some undone business. Examples would be someone with whom they are angry with or wish to say something special to. They are asked to raise a finger if they can visualise someone sitting in the chair. Volunteers are asked to talk about it and perhaps approach the person and have something to say. Group members must never be forced to participate.

The group member can also go and sit in the chair and assume the position of the person they have visualised and talk about it from there.

This is an excellent technique for group members to release their anxiety, to resolve issues and conflicts and also to have the opportunity to say important things to a person in a safe environment. They can literally 'let off steam'. The use of a 'Baticar', a small softly stuffed doll can be very useful to smack a person without hurting them. This is easily made by an occupational therapist (Figure 9.2).

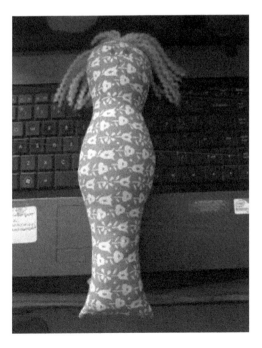

FIGURE 9.2 The baticar which is just a stuffed toy. It is easy to hit someone with it without causing damage.

9.12   WARM-UPS WHICH INCLUDE SOME PHYSICAL CONTACT

Warm-up techniques are mostly used to get group members physically active in some way in a group (see the contribution by Louise Fouché). Using techniques where group members are in physical contact also usually fosters close relationships in a group. Be warned however that some religions do not allow physical contact between the sexes and also that some group members may be tactile defensive. In the author's experience tactile methods quite often foster love or sexual relationships too.

Examples of these techniques are:

- Blind walk where a group member is blindfolded and has to identify fellow members by feeling and touching them. This is conducted by the group leader who helps the group member experience textures, small shapes and sounds. On identification of the person, a discussion ensues.
- The trust game where a group member closes his/her eyes and is allowed to fall against a tightly closed group. Group members catch the group member at the back on the scapulas. The persons are handed over to another group member physically. This is excellent to develop trust and cohesiveness in the group.
- Crossing over hands in a closed group and then untangling into an open group.
- Some of the techniques described in the carousel such as holding hands and feeling each other's faces with eyes shut.

9.13   THE USE OF HAND PUPPETS OR MASKS

Puppets can be used as an introduction but can also be used as an entire psychodrama with group members playing the role of the puppet. For a warm-up, the group member introduces him/herself through the puppet. Masks can be used in the same way. Often this is the start of a very interesting occupational group therapy session and is highly recommended. Hand puppets can easily be made in an occupational therapy activity group session but blowing up a balloon and covering it with papiere maché and moulded to resemble a desired face. When dry the balloon is removed and the face painted and varnished. The body part is sewn on.

Masks can also be made out of papiere maché in the same way.

9.14 JOHARI'S WINDOW

Finally the author would like to recommend a book entitled 'Gamester's Hand Book Two' written by Donna Brandes in 1982. It contains many ideas for warm-up including the Johari's Window which is often used. Johari's window which is four squares like a window is drawn on a piece of paper by each group member. In one square is written 'Things that others know about me', in the second window 'Things about me that others know and I don't', the third window 'Things I know others don't know about me', and the fourth window 'Things that no-one knows about me'. In this book are three examples of assertiveness warm-ups and many other excellent examples.

Other warm-up techniques may be invented by the occupational therapist to increase social interaction and emotional interaction in occupational group therapy. Often music is played to relax or stimulate emotion and also verbal interaction. Once again it is a creative process and occupational therapists are experts at these interventions. It is an essential part of any group and gradually develops involvement of each group member.

CHAPTER 10

Role-play

'Role play is an experiential way of teaching and learning skills (Nove 1989. p. B79). It is one of the most effective teaching methods that exists and in occupational therapy is often used as part of group work, particularly when social skills training is taking place. Role-play is a task-centred procedure that is used to teach people to play roles in life and to solve their problems. It is, however, not psychodrama!

When comparing psychodrama and role-play Blatner (1973) states that 'Most professionals would consider role-playing to be more superficial and problem-orientated' (p. 10). There might be some emotional involvement but evoking emotions is not the purpose of the exercise and should be kept to a minimum. As stated by Blatner (1973), the goal of role-playing tends to be working out alternative and more effective approaches to a general problem and is a tool for bringing about specific behaviour and its effect into focus.

Role-play can be carried out in individual therapy but is obviously more effective in a group where there are people to play roles and more people to learn. Situations such as interviews for jobs, confrontations, stressful situations such as taking a rotten bag of oranges back

Occupational Group Therapy, First Edition. Rosemary Crouch.

to a shop and getting your money back are typical examples. Role-play is used in industry, in business and in the training of health professionals. It is also used as an integral part in the training in assertiveness and stress management. It is a vital part of social skills training particularly with clients with intellectual disabilities who need to practise the most effective way of communicating with others. A disabled person will often ask 'what do I say after I have said hello.'

It must be noted that participants in role-play can feel vulnerable; it therefore requires that the group leader provides a safe structure and needs to be quite directive (Bundey et al. 1984). Setting up the venue for role-play is important but does not have to be highly structured as in psychodrama. It should take place where everyone in the group can see the interaction and volunteers are usually used as fellow role-players. Role-players must be voluntary but can often be suggested by the group leader. They should be carefully put into their roles and never demanded to play a role. This process is called 'enrolling'.

When the goal of the group has been made clear to the group members a few tables and chairs are moved into position, either inside the group or at the side. Props such as a telephone, a desk pad and pencil and a bottle and glass can be useful.

The occupational group therapist then helps the group members establish what the real situation is and assists in structuring the role-play. A situation can be acted out many times, with different or the same people, until a level of competency is achieved. A discussion ensues and the group members have time to discuss their reaction to the role-play and how they felt playing the role.

Humour and laughing always make the situation fun and usually group members thoroughly enjoy the role-play and remember it for a long time afterwards.

It is always essential to de-role participants before the group ends, because often group members enjoy, or get stuck in a role and continue to play it outside of the group. The author uses two methods of de-roling:

1. Ask the group members to state clearly his/her own name and who he/she is not, e.g. 'I am Mary and not the director of the company'!

2. Ask the role-players to brush the role they have been playing off themselves with large brushes on the side of their body with their hands. At the same time they say clearly their own names and that they are not the person whose role they have been playing.

Occupational group therapists should be aware that at any time a group member playing a role may want to stop. He/she should always be allowed to do this. It should be noted also that the whole role-play can be stopped if it is in anyway getting out of hand, or that the occupational therapist feels out of control.

Case Study 1:   Role-play Used with Young School-Going Boys

The author, occupational group therapist, was asked to set up a group with six 12- to 13-year-old boys who were the sons of professionals with whom she worked. They were 'normal' children who had issues such a bullying at school, seemingly unfair judgements by teachers, how to deal with disciplinary action, issues with other boys at school such as the way they responded to teachers etc.
The aims of this group were:

- To develop self-esteem in the handling of everyday issues at school and social development.
- To share similar problems with other boys of their own age.
- To have an opportunity to share these problems in a safe environment, that is alternative to the home environment.
- To develop skills in handling problems in a controlled manner and in a way that is socially appropriate.

The group took place after-school in a group room in a house where the occupational therapy practice was located. It took place once a week, for one hour, for six weeks. Cool drinks and snacks were provided for the start of the group only.

The group set their own norms, guided by the occupational group therapist. These norms were:

- No cell phones on or used during the group.
- No eating.
- Bad language to a minimum.
- No leaving the group before the closure unless to the toilet.

Role-play was the most frequent technique used during the group process and was extremely effective. The boys took to the technique very quickly and not only enjoyed playing their own role in order to get the problem off their minds, but loved playing the role of the Head Master, the bully, etc. It was almost as if they were getting their own back.

The venue was quite structured with items such as a desk and chairs, a telephone and a door which could be shut and knocked upon. Role identification was dealt with promptly when a group member offered to play a role.

The group watched from a close distance. They were asked their opinions and often to play a role that they had commented on.

It was extremely successful. There were silent and intense moments and much laughter and enjoyment. Feedback from parents indicated that experiential learning of skills had taken place and much enjoyment.

Case Study 2:   Training of Community Rehabilitation/ Health Workers using Role-play as a Technique

The handling of residents in a rural community who suffer from mental illness is a very difficult and sensitive issue. The author experienced the training of Community Rehabilitation Workers (CRWs) and used role-play as the major technique of training. Practical handling of community members is required and therefore lecturing to caring people with different educational backgrounds on issues such as handling people with mental conditions is not easy. Lectures, unless very pictorial and with videos, are not appropriate. From experience the workers do not retain the information from lectures or written notes. Experience was much more successful.

Role-play is without a doubt the most successful technique to teach the realities of various conditions found in people who live in an impoverished community and also to teach handling and treatment techniques to workers in a practical way that will 'stick'. The use of role-play is best in a group because there are group members to call upon to play roles.

In this instance the aims of using role-play were:

- Educational in an active way rather than by lectures or written notes.
- Experiential, so that the roles students played are practised and familiar.
- The roles people played, especially as the client/patient had been observed previously and were authentic.
- The experience of cohesive group work where students could trust one another.

Setting up the role-play should be quite formal although the author has observed spontaneous role-play in a group just where people were sitting and it was very effective.

Chairs and tables should be set apart from the rest of the group and often useful extras are a telephone, a bottle of water and glass, a notebook pad and pencil. Other professional equipment such as a wheelchair, walker, etc. may be necessary.

The training of participants in their roles is not as important as it is in psychodrama. Usually group members are eager to volunteer for a role such as the shopkeeper, the boss, the teacher or a parent.

The role-play can then take place for as long as it takes. Swapping over of roles occurs when a group member says 'oh no this is what you should have said/done'. The occupational group therapist then asks the group member to 'have a go' at that role. The role-play repeats.

CHAPTER 11

The Use of Psychodrama and the Therapeutic Spiral Model in Occupational Group Therapy

In 1975 a very interesting article was published in the British Journal of Occupational Therapy by (Mclean 1975, p. 163). As an occupational therapist she had the privilege of training as a psychodramatist at the Moreno Institute in New York. She wrote a very interesting article called 'An encounter: Occupational therapy and psychodrama'. She asked the question 'how does one profession compliment the other? What similarities, if any, are there between the two professions? How can knowledge of psychodramatic theory assist the occupational therapist?' Without a doubt this was really the start of occupational therapists becoming involved in the use of psychodramatic techniques and many occupational therapists all over the world are now using these techniques in their occupational group therapy.

In the author's opinion is it is not a case of changing profession but using very valuable techniques taken from their training in psychodrama, in their own occupational group therapy. Louise Fouché (Chapter 2) and Vivyan Alers (to whom this book is dedicated, who used the Therapeutic Spiral psychodramatic techniques) and the author all trained extensively in the psychodramatic techniques in South Africa, England and France.

Howard Blatner (1973) stated that 'Psychodrama is a method whereby a person can be helped to explore the psychological dimension of his problems through the enactment of his conflict situations, rather than talking about them' (p. 6). Psychodrama refers to an enactment involving emotional problem-solving and is essentially a systemised method of acting out within the confines of a close cohesive group. 'Psychodrama is a method of group therapy in which patients enact the relevant events in their lives instead of simply talking about them. Psychodrama can refer to both a specific therapeutic method and also the use of a wider variety of techniques that have application in therapy, business, education, as well as in many other areas' (Blatner 1973, p. 2).

This form of group therapy is concerned with the acting out of one person's problem or conflict during the group process. The other members of the group may co-act with the group member concerned and help him/her explore the problem or just observe from a position in the group and become involved through identification with the group members who are involved in the group process. Psychodrama is a very powerful tool and all the dynamics of a close cohesive group come very much into play. It seems that the actual movement and activity enhance the group involvement and if used correctly can be a very therapeutic process in any group therapy.

In psychodrama, drama is used in a spontaneous way in individual, family and group settings. Moreno (1946) stated that 'Psychodrama can be defined therefore, as the science which explores the truth by dramatic methods'.

Group members can learn to develop spontaneity, creativity and self-disclosure through action. They also learn the importance of the present which is referred to as the 'here-and-now'. This is a term which was coined by Jacob Moreno, the father of psychodrama in 1946. Other important aspects of psychodrama is the understanding of the significance of touch and nonverbal communication, thereby cultivating imagination and intuition through the depth of drama. It is interesting to note that one of the most valuable dynamics of psychodrama is that the technique demonstrates the value of humour.

In 1911 Jacob Moreno was a medical student in Vienna. He watched children playing and acted as a catalyst encouraging them to act out spontaneously in dramatic role-play. From 1921 to 1923 Moreno started the 'Theatre of Spontaneity' (Das Stegreif Theatre). He took his work to America in 1925 and founded the Moreno Institute, with his wife Zerka. He died in 1974 and Zerka carried on his work.

The other members of the group co-act with the person concerned and help him explore his problem or just observe it from the group and often become involved through identification.

Like many other specialised techniques, psychodrama is not taught in any depth at undergraduate level in occupational therapy programmes in the world. In most occupational therapy courses psychodrama is mentioned and training in psychodrama has been available at a postgraduate level. The methods can be modified and used in many occupational therapy group settings. It is a very powerful tool and all the dynamics of a close cohesive group come into play. If one looks at the integral part action and activity have in the very definition of occupational therapy, it is obvious that this type of drama is going to meet the scope of the occupational therapy profession in most countries.

A letter received in 1973 from Zerka Moreno, wife of Jacob Moreno, states that psychodrama is not a technique confined to any one profession. Blatner (1988) provides a long list of professionals for which psychodrama is particularly suitable, e.g. creative arts therapists who want to integrate psychodrama with art, poetry, music, dance and the like; 'people helpers', including nurses, social workers, leaders of self-help groups, and recreation workers.

One of the most famous psychodramatists in the world is an occupational therapist, Gillie Ruskombe-King, who is a contributor to one of the famous books to ever be written on Psychodrama by Holmes et al. (1994).

For many years occupational therapists all over the world have been using projective techniques such as drama, art and music as part of their group therapy and also with the individual patient. These techniques fall very well into the scope of the profession, especially as they are so creative in nature.

Psychodrama is not an analytical or interpretative technique. These processes fall into the scope of psychologists not occupational therapists, but it requires knowledge and expertise to be effective. It must be structured correctly and emotions are not the main focus of attention.

Psychodrama must be carried out by a well-trained professional whose training has been incorporated through practical and theoretical training in group work.

Usually the training takes place at postgraduate level. It is not a technique that should be used by a layperson or untrained volunteer. Moreno (1946) stated that the psychodramatist should be able to 'impress the group with the importance of the work'. A good sense of humour and sense of fun is a definite asset. Knowledge of the theatre and being able to act is not important. Obviously the occupational therapist must have developed insight into self, relationships, behaviour, etc.

What are the benefits of using this technique? There are many which include:

- Relief of anxiety. It is actually relaxation in action!
- Reality testing.
- Channelisation and expression of anger in a controlled setting.
- Behavioral change.
- Stimulation of emotional response and psychomotor stimulation.
- Assertiveness training.
- Motivation for additional therapy.

The major players in this type of group therapy are:

- The director or psychodramatist (the group leader): This is the person who guides the group through the process of the psychodramatic method. It must be a trained professional.
- The group: Group members must be thoroughly assessed beforehand and skilfully placed in the group. They must agree

to participate and due to lack of trust may ask the group leader if they can attend without participating. This should be allowed because very often, due to the nature of the group, this client will get caught up in the interaction. Group members will be dictated by the diagnosis or the setting and definitely by their level of creative participation and functional ability. Sometimes group members are excluded because of psychosis, hypomania and severe personality disorders such as borderline disorders. Professional actors/actresses often disrupt the psychodrama because they tend to exaggerate roles and are able to mask their real role in life. 8–10 group members are ideal.

- The protagonist: This person is the subject of the psychodramatic enactment who presents the problem or difficult situation. It may be a problem in the past, present or future. There is only one protagonist in classic psychodrama. The protagonist comes to light in the group by volunteering spontaneously or may have agreed to present his/her problem previously. He/she may be chosen by the group after the warm-up or may just emerge from the warm-up exercise. The protagonist should not be chosen by the group leader and forced to participate.

- The auxiliary (ego): This is the significant co-actor who is chosen by the protagonist. They are often mothers, fathers, siblings, bosses, friends, etc. who help the protagonist explore the problem. It is possible for the group leader to appoint a professional auxiliary.

- A system of methods and techniques adaptable to the requirements of the situation – the process of psychodrama.

The group must have a chance to develop cohesiveness before the psychodrama takes place. Therefore three or four group sessions are recommended to take place before the introduction of psychodrama.

- The warm-up (see Chapter 9): It is extremely important to carry out a warm-up at the commencement of psychodrama as acting out can appear to be quite threatening and often the anxiety level of the group members is high at the commencement. Feelings of 'what am I going to be expected to do' are common. The warm-up stimulates interaction and during this time the protagonist is often identified.

- The action: When the protagonist has been determined by the group and is ready to work, the exploration of the problem begins. The protagonist is given time to briefly discuss the problem and set the scene. Often this procedure is bypassed if the protagonist is already in the position where spontaneous action can take place after the warm-up. In this case the other group members are asked to sit back in the group and the action begins.

Setting the scene: It is extremely important to give the protagonist time to set up the most realistic scene possible with the available furniture etc. The psychodramatist should walk around the scene with the psychodramatist describing the physical layout as well as the feelings that the scene engenders.

The problem is then redefined for the sake of the whole group and the selection of auxiliary egos takes place. It is important for the protagonist to select all auxiliary egos as previously described except where a double (see the next section on definable psychodrama techniques) is required. The double is often selected by the psychodramatist, as skill is often required for this purpose. The protagonist then describes the roles to the auxiliary egos and role reversal can be used here, two or three times, for the protagonist to demonstrate the behaviour of him/his co-actors. The drama then begins and the problem presented in dramatic form.

The act completion can occur in a number of ways. It may result in catharsis. In this case, it is best, where possible, to come back into the security of the group where the protagonist can safely let go. If not, the psychodramatist firmly supports the protagonist in situ. Sometimes very sympathetic group members may approach the protagonist a hug or create some closeness. (See below the Section 11.1.)

The action may just come to an end or the psychodramatist may immediately start to alter the scene.

There are definable psychodrama techniques that are used during the action. Those most commonly used are

- Self-presentation: This is the basic, straight forward most commonly used psychodramatic technique. The protagonist depicts his own situation as it is in the 'here-and-now', even though it may have elements of the past or future. 'He shows how people behave and what is said and not said; and, using various basic dramatic techniques, he portrays his own phenomenological and psychodramatic world plays his own psychodramatic world' (Blatner 1988, p. 175).
- Role reversal: Role reversal is one of the most effective ways of encouraging the protagonist to see him/herself through the eyes of others.

  Role reversal has two purposes. The first is when the protagonist instructs the auxiliary egos as to their roles at the start and setting up of the psychodrama. It is a form of role training. The protagonist switches roles with the auxiliary ego and in doing so demonstrates how the other person behaves. It assists greatly in making the enactment as real as possible. This technique can also be employed in role-play. The protagonist can role reverse with as many auxiliaries as he/she thinks necessary.

  The second purpose of role reversal is when it is used later on in the enactment when it is desirable for the protagonist to look at the situation from the position of another person. In this way he/she may develop insights into both his/her own behaviour or the other person's situation. This assists in choosing more adaptive responses. 'Role-reversal is indicated when it is appropriate for the protagonist to empathize with the other person's point of view' (Blatner 1988, p. 175). 'Thus, role reversal becomes a major technique for building the capacity for empathy with others' (Blatner 1973, p. 73).

  It is important to note that the auxiliary ego in the role reversal does not have to resemble the protagonist at all.

  Soliloquy (similar to the Shakespearian soliloquy): Using this technique requires the protagonist to 'go it alone'. This means that he/she can work through difficulties without any interference by others. It is a spontaneous process and is encouraged by the psychodramatist walking around with him/her at a slight distance encouraging continuation of the process. It is also a highly effective technique which is often preferred by the protagonist.

- The double: This technique is often termed 'the heart of psychodrama'. An auxiliary ego or group member, chosen by the protagonist or suggested by the psychodramatist, stands just behind the protagonist, often with a hand on his/her shoulder. The double should assume a similar pose to the protagonist. The double is often termed the alter ego and is both support and encouragement to the protagonist. As with role reversal, the double does not have to resemble the protagonist at all.

    This process engenders good expression and dialogue. The double suggests to the protagonist words that could be used to make the altercation or communication more effective. The double should not talk directly to the other person to whom the protagonist is talking, only to the protagonist.

    This technique is used as a way to encourage a shy person to say what he/she has on he/his mind, to help express emotions like anger and love, and to gain confidence. It stimulates interaction and empathy.

    A double can also be used in the technique of soliloquy.

    From experience one knows that if the double encourages the protagonist to say something that is not in his/her mind, the protagonist will not respond, or will say to the double 'that is not what I am feeling'.

- Future projection: This technique allows the protagonist to project him/herself into the future and to shape and explore some of the other dimensions of his situation. He may gain a more realistic approach and begin to portray scenes in which he can achieve successes based on his own work. The protagonist is given time to briefly discuss the problem in the group before being asked by the psychodramatist to set the scene. Often this procedure is bypassed if the protagonist is already in a position where a spontaneous action can take place after the warm-up. In this case the other group members are asked to sit back in the group and the action begins.

- The empty chair (auxiliary chair): An empty chair is used instead of an auxiliary ego. This could lead to a more spontaneous expression of emotions and is very powerful.

  An empty chair is placed in the middle of the group and members are asked if they can visualise someone sitting in the chair with whom they have some undone business or someone they would like to express something to. This technique can be used as a warm-up but the chair can also be used as a significant other in the psychodrama. The group member is asked to stand up or sit and address the chair, encouraged by the psychodramatist. If the group member feels angry they may kick the chair which he/she would not be able to do if it was a person. The empty chair can also be used in the enactment if there is not a suitable auxiliary ego and this is often used in the warm-up technique of sculpting (see Chapter 9).

- The mirror: In this technique the protagonist sits back and watches an auxiliary ego represent himself/herself. It is similar to role reversal. However, in the author's experience, as the protagonist instructs the auxiliary ego, frustration usually prevails and the protagonist is soon back in his/her original position. It is a way of encouraging a protagonist who is reluctant to act out.

11.1   THE INTEGRATION AND PROCESSING

The psychodramatist now directs the group into the working through phase. This is called the integration or processing.

Sometimes, particularly when the protagonist is very emotional, the working through consists of sharing and discussion with the group and no more action takes place.

If a catharsis, which is usually on the part of the protagonist but also may be a group member, has taken place or when there is just act-completion, the psychodramatist uses his/her skills to introduce various techniques to help the protagonist work through the problem. The techniques of role reversal, repeating and trying out a situation, acting out of anger, confrontation, etc. takes place here. This is where the empty chair can be effectively used again.

When some realisation or relief has occurred the group members come back to the group together and sharing takes place. The protagonist always needs much support at this stage and it is wise for the psychodramatist to sit as close as possible to the protagonist.

When the group members share they must be directed into sharing their feelings rather than their feeling on how the protagonist can solve the problem. Fouché in Section 3.1 makes this very clear. The identification of the problem for each group member will then come to the fore and this process is of great value to them, in identifying with the protagonist's problem the group members inadvertently support the protagonist in what she/he has shared with the group.

Discussion then takes place during which time the director must be assured by the protagonist that she/he is comfortable enough in what has been shared before terminating the group. If not, the group must be patient in allowing the protagonist to get everything off her/his chest.

11.2   THE CLOSURE AN ESSENTIAL PROCESS IN PSYCHODRAMA INCLUDING THE DE-ROLING

De-roling is a very important procedure. Each group member who has played a role, and the protagonist, must be given an opportunity to discuss with the group how they felt playing the role and the significance in his/her life. The group member is asked to say, e.g. I am 'Jo Blogs and not Jim Smith'. Role-players are often asked to physically brush themselves off to demonstrate this de-roling. Occupational group therapists must be aware of the fact that playing a role can be important and that a group member may take this role out of the group and continue playing it!

Closure must be final and complete before the end of the group and the protagonist and auxiliaries acknowledged. Many psychodramatists clap their hands and stand up to finalise the group. A really potent end to the group is to stand and wave and say goodbye (this is an international practice and highly recommended!).

Often the protagonist sits quietly alone with the occupational therapist after the group to consolidate what has taken place as a supportive measure. Occupational therapists who have the privilege of working in a close professional team will discuss the interaction during psychodrama with the protagonist's individual therapist.

Case Study: A Long-Term Community Group with Women and Men Who Are Recovering Alcoholics, Using Psychodrama on a Frequent Basis

A strong, versatile group of 8–10 men and women, mostly middle-aged alcoholics (also with other substance use disorders) came together in 1993 in a private practice in Johannesburg for more than 19 years. The original group evolved from people who had been discharged from a rehabilitation centre outside Johannesburg and needed an aftercare group. Some were referred by social workers, psychologists and psychiatrists or general practitioners. Most of the group members also attended Alcoholics Anonymous (the AA or NAD). The group therapist/psychodramatist was an occupational therapist trained in psychodrama and all group members were assessed by her before being introduced to the group. All clients had to be functioning on the level of Active Participation and above (VdTMoCA 2019) before being accepted for the group.

The aims of the group were as follows:

- Maintenance of sobriety was the main aim: All group members were expected to be 'clean'. There were a few occasions where a group member arrived who had been drinking and had tried to cover it up with masses of cologne or peppermints but was quickly diagnosed and confronted by the group. The group member was not asked to leave because of the danger of he/she feeling rejected, but was dealt with by the group members directed by the occupational group therapist. Psychodrama is the most potent technique on an occasion like this and is a very therapeutic measure. Usually the intervention is effective.

- Developing self-esteem and confidence: Having the opportunity to be the central part of an enactment in psychodrama as a group member, supported by the psychodramatist, is a life-changing experience. Whether it is a soliloquy or a full enactment with auxiliary egos to interact with the protagonist, it is an experience not to be forgotten. One of the most powerful reasons is that it takes place actively and is in the 'here-and-now'. It is happening now and it lasts! There is absolutely no doubt that the group members developed self-esteem and confidence and that this led to many years of sobriety and a better life.
- Improving relationships: Relationships become severely damaged through the excessive use of alcohol and other drugs. Marriages break up and other good relationships damaged. Psychodrama used in this way defines the path to restore these relationships and helps to bring realisation into how new and old relationships can be built again. The whole process of psychodrama is one of the best techniques to explore this process. And try them out in the action. A sense of happiness and contentment can be the result. Of course, this is extremely important when a group member is battling with an addiction.
- Substitution for the addiction: From an occupational therapy point of view, an addict needs to build a new life that includes increased occupational performance and the participation in new activities and interests, and very often psychodrama can lead the way in this respect. New avenues and ideas open and group members support each other in these issues.

The group met once a week after work at 17h00 and the group could last up to two hours. The venue was easily accessible by car, taxi or bus and most group members were from the middle socioeconomic income group and spoke English, or sometimes Afrikaans or an African language such as Zulu. All of them understood English which was the language of the group. There were a variety of cultures and religions amongst the members which made the group very interesting. Some examples are Zulu, Sotho, Jewish, Christian South African, Italian Roman Catholic and English. This made for an excellent heterogeneous group which developed a strong cohesiveness over a period of time even though there were obvious changes as members came and went during the years. There was always a core of group members.

A warm-up technique was always used at the beginning of the group and the most popular techniques were the cards, the magic shop, sculpting and the empty chair. Because of the high level of cohesiveness the group members became very used to psychodrama and knew what to expect. Consequently there was very little difficulty in finding a protagonist. If a protagonist was not identified in a group session then the occupational group therapist would change the direction of the group and a discussion and sometimes relaxation would take place instead. Sometimes role-play was used where there was no emotional, or very little, emotional involvement. The protagonist from a psychodrama would often stay behind for a while to consolidate and for the occupational therapists to be sure he/she was in a state to go home. The person's personal counsellor was often contacted the next day by the occupational therapist to be informed of the developments. The client was informed of this.

Issues that were acted out in the psychodrama often revolved around relationships, the actual addiction process which often included times when the client was tempted to drink again or did actually relapse, loss of jobs, loss of friends, etc. It was very seldom that a group member was chosen by the occupational therapist who did not fit in.

Most of the group members remained well during this period. If they relapsed, they quickly 'got back onto the wagon' again with the help of the group. It was extremely successful and highly recommended.

11.3   THE THERAPEUTIC SPIRAL TECHNIQUE OF PSYCHODRAMA (VIVYAN ALERS)

The Therapeutic Spiral Model is a technique of psychodrama described by Hudgens (2002). Vivyan Alers was an expert in the Therapeutic Spiral Technique and was trained internationally. Included under this heading is a transcript from her chapter in 'Occupational Therapy: An African Perspective' for which she was chief editor with Rosemary Crouch (2010).

This technique or model was developed primarily for use with trauma survivors. Vivyan Alers worked in an impoverished township near Pretoria in South Africa where she used this technique very successfully with a group of impoverished and traumatised young people. Typical traumas involved women and child abuse, violence, deprivation, clashes with the law, accidents, etc., either experienced or observed.

'The Therapeutic Spiral Model always begins with building strengths to resource the self to prevent re-traumatisation. Safety and containment are key components of this model. The person chooses three scarves or pieces of material, to represent his/her personal, interpersonal and transpersonal (spiritual) strengths. The colours, textures or patterns represent aspects of life, which are meaningful to the person. These strengths are seen as the person's roles and this process ensures that at any one time more "positive" roles are present than "negative" roles. Again these strengths are discussed in pairs and then within the group where the strengths are presented individually and placed on the floor to form a "community circle of safety". The group symbolically breathing in the strength does acknowledgement of each of the strengths. These strengths are called the prescriptive roles. The circle of scarves is also the containment circle. The containment concept is to enable the individual not to become overwhelmed or feel uncontrollably vulnerable especially when emotional flooding occurs. It establishes a "safe" place to work through experiences in the "here and now" (Moreno 1975). The occupational therapist also chooses his or her own strengths and shares this with a partner. This is also a method of combatting compassion fatigue. This model is based on three strands of the spiral: building energy, providing experience and making meaning of the experience' (p. 278, Chapter 14).

CHAPTER 12

Life-Skills Cognitive-Behavioural Groups, Assertiveness Training Groups and Social Skills Training (Verbal and Nonverbal) Groups

12.1 INTRODUCTION

There are a number of well-known occupational therapy experts on the subject of life-skills such as Creek and Lougher (2008) who state that 'Life skills enable people to operate as individuals and contribute to them functioning as part of society in which they belong' (p. 360).

Roberts (2008) in the same publication states that 'Psycho-social life skills are a group of skills based on behaviour, cognition and interaction. Affective and anxiety disorders may be associated with life-skill deficits which become the focus of occupational

Occupational Group Therapy, First Edition. Rosemary Crouch.
© 2021 John Wiley & Sons Ltd. Published 2021 by John Wiley & Sons Ltd.

therapy intervention in order to enable the client to function at an optimal level' (pp. 364–368).

One of the most successful publications on this subject is that of Wilkinson and Canter (1982). This still remains the best practical and informative book on the subject of social skills and is a manual which is very practical and highly recommended.

A cognitive-behavioural approach is required for all of these training groups and the occupational therapist must be well versed in these skills techniques before attempting them. Usually this is at undergraduate level but skills can be developed in well-planned postgraduate training groups.

12.2   ASSERTIVENESS TRAINING

Assertiveness training is a social skills technique employed by a number of health professionals and there is much literature available. This training can be presented individually or in a group. This chapter will only address assertiveness training within occupational group therapy. Clearly this does not have to be a technique that is only used in a clinical setting. Other professionals and occupational therapists working with lifestyle training in companies and in various work places as well as educational institutions are using this technique.

In this instance however, since it is part of therapy, we are talking about occupational group therapy both in a hospital or a community setting. It is appropriate in both, but with clients/patients who are functioning at the level of active participation (at least) according to the VdTMoC (van der Reyden et al. 2019).

Occupational therapy paradigms are primarily based on the concepts of occupational performance and occupational engagement as a means of promoting health and well-being. (WFOT 2002). A small group setting in the occupational therapy programme is ideal for assertiveness training. Occupational therapists have the right kind of background and training to develop expertise in this field. A life-skill such as assertiveness deals directly with the everyday occupations of people because it has to do with the ability to relate effectively in many different situations, at home, at work and social settings. The success of many occupations depends on the ability to communicate, to express deeply held personal values, social conditioning, feelings of self-esteem, peer expectations and cultural influences (Nove 1984).

A small group of approximately eight people is most successful because it 'creates an atmosphere where participants feel accepted, at ease, free to express doubts and to challenge new information and to practise skills - without fear of judgement or ridicule' (Nove 1984).

It is important to state at the outset that cultural values and issues must be recognised, especially when working in a multicultural setting with a subject like assertiveness. When working in the community the occupational therapist must be familiar with the cultural values of that particular area, particularly in South Africa where there are so many different cultures. Even today it is not appropriate for a woman to stand up for or disagree with her husband in some cultures – however this does not mean that she cannot learn to be appropriately assertive and retain or improve her self-esteem (see Section 5.5. on cultural considerations).

Learning to be assertive cannot be done by reading a written handout from the occupational therapist. Once again it must be stressed that it is an active technique. Icebreaker and warm-up techniques are appropriate and role-play is integral to teaching someone to be assertive (see Chapter 9). Feedback and sharing are vital to the group. How often one hears a group member say 'okay if you don't think I'm any good at it, you come and show me how'!

12.3   BASIC CONCEPTS

How does one define the term assertive? Perhaps it is easiest to say what it is not!:

- It is not aggression. Aggression is winning by humiliation, degrading, belittling or overpowering the other person. From a relationship point of view, the aggressive person always loses. Aggression always violates the rights of the other person.

- A person who is unassertive violates his/her own rights because of a failure to stand up for her/himself! Others often disregard the person especially the person who is always apologising. However the person who can apologise assertively is always held in high regard.

Being assertive involves the following:

- Assertive behaviour 'is a natural style that is nothing more than being direct, honest, and respectful while interacting with others' (Lloyd 1988).
- Expressing one's thoughts, feelings and beliefs in a direct, honest and appropriate way at the right time. The motto is: 'This is what I think, this is how I feel and this is how I see the situation'. Examples are: 'What you are saying to me is very rude, I feel violated and think you should go and take out your anger with the punch bag at the gym'. Or 'I think it is wonderful what you are saying, it makes me feel really good and I see a real future in our working together'. It is standing up for yourself and your rights. It is all said without dominating, humiliating or degrading the other person. It is a win-win situation.
- Nonverbal communication is very important. It is difficult to be assertive when you are looking aggressive or looking downtrodden. Stand up straight, put your shoulders back, if appropriate culturally, look the person straight in the eye!

Please see Appendix B for detailed information and well-tried material used in assertiveness training.

12.3.1　Social Skills Training

Much information in this section is derived from Wilkinson and Canter (1982). This publication gives excellent examples of social skills training programmes.

Social skills training groups are often employed during broader training programmes and are very definitely most effective when carried out in groups. It should be noted however that social skills training can also be carried out on a one-to-one basis. Occupational therapists are absolute experts from their training in the leading of these groups, as good skills in leading groups are required and they are also trained in techniques such as role-play and warm-up techniques.

Examples of the type of person that social skills training groups are appropriate with are people with chronic psychiatric disorders, persons with one of the spectrum of autistic disorders, intellectually handicapped people, disturbed adolescents and sometimes with offenders in institutions. Assertiveness is also a social skill but is kept separate in this book as assertiveness training it is most usually performed with people who are functioning at the level of Active Participation (VdTMoCA 2019) or higher. See the previous chapter for details on assertiveness training.

Social skills which would be introduced during comprehensive multidisciplinary programmes are subjects suitable for group work. Issues such as these below are usually the subject of the occupational group therapy:

Nonverbal skills which include (Wilkinson and Canter 1982):

- Posture, gait, personal distance and gesture.
- Facial expression, eye contact, vocal cues and tone of voice.

Verbal behaviour such as:

- Listening, encouraging the other to talk and asking questions (p. 85).
- Greetings, talking and maintaining conversation, opening and closing conversations.

Topics that are often used as subject in the social skills groups are:

- Sharing, such as giving a present, or receiving it.
- Showing something of interest to someone else such as a new mobile phone.

- Going to the shop and buying something of the group member's choice. In this case you can include two or three group members, two people shopping together and one shopkeeper (the magic shop warm-up technique is very good here but used in a concrete sense rather than emotional).
- Taking back damaged or unacceptable produce you have bought to the shop.
- Taking and giving messages.
- Applying for a job and job interviews.
- Asking for a raise in salary.
- Coping with bullying and harassment.
- Telling someone you really like them or love them.
- Praising someone for something they have done.
- Disclosing displeasure with something that has happened.
- Approaching someone that has offended you.

The actual group process proceeds according to all the guidelines given for occupational group therapy in the previous chapters. The group must be developed and run professionally with assessment of the participants, the venue properly prepared, the aims of the group set, preparation of the participants with each one knowing what they are in the group for and the aims, the group introduction, procedure and firm closure with the reiteration of the aims which group and individuals have achieved. This is delightful and very concrete and successful intervention. It is a very good way for occupational therapy students to learn group work.

CHAPTER 13

Community-Based Stress Management with Emphasis on Group Work

This chapter addresses stress management with particular reference to community work. In most rural and urban communities, there can be a lack of professional health professionals particularly in the middle- and lower income groups and in countries where poverty and hardship abound. Group work is the obvious choice in order to spread the advantage of professional intervention which in this chapter addresses stress management.

Research indicates that living in poverty increases stress, which leads to a greater risk of mental health difficulties both for children and for adults

Turnbull (2002).

Ritchie (1970) stated 'Although not conclusively proven, stress is implicated as a risk factor in the most common causes of disease and death' (p. 7). Stress management is one of those techniques

Occupational Group Therapy, First Edition. Rosemary Crouch.

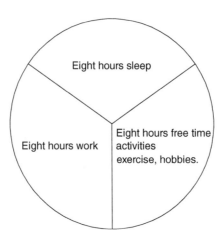

FIGURE 13.1   A 24-hour balanced lifestyle divisions: sleep, work and play.

frequently used in occupational therapy that is particularly suitable for group work and most essential in the community. The very nature of the occupational therapist is the trained ability to be versatile and provide a holistic approach to intervention. Stress management embraces most aspects of one's daily life from waking up in the morning to going to sleep at night. Stress management principles apply to a balance of daily activity which is ideally eight hours of sleep, eight hours of work and eight hours of play/relaxing activity/ personal interests (Figure 13.1).

The models of occupational therapy address occupational performance, and the ability to handle stress in every sphere of life is considered central. The ever-increasing stress factors in the environment include economic, political factors, an increase in the pace of life, fast cars, fast-foods, unemployment, etc.

In 2008 Crouch developed and evaluated a programme for the effective management of stress in an impoverished rural community in South Africa. This study addresses the destructive stress that abounds in and challenges the impoverished people who live in rural areas of South Africa, where the majority of the country's population is located. Poverty and the accompanying problems, as proved by Crouch in her research, can be influenced by semi-structured group work embracing stress management at meeting spots in the community such as local clinics and church halls. The results of her research show that certain stress management programmes are suitable for community groups (in particular a South African community in this case). The results could be generalised to other impoverished communities (See the next section 13.1).

13.1 WHAT IS STRESS?

'Stress is the response of the body to physical and/or psychological demands made on it by events, changes or circumstances. These demands may emanate from the internal or external environment and tax or exceed the adaptive or coping capacity of an individual' (R. B. Crouch, unpublished manual). It consists of:

1. The stressor, the changes or demands.
2. How this stressor is perceived.
3. The actual stress response in the body or the mind.

Stress means different things to different people. One person's stressors can be another person's fun. In other words, people react differently to situations according to their physical, emotional and intellectual makeup. If the occupational therapist compares the stress factors in life in an impoverished community to that of life in an affluent business community in a city, stress factors differ.

In the rural community, three stress management techniques was found by Crouch (2008) to be suitable for group work in this community. All three groups took place once a week for four weeks and were followed up after eight weeks. The most effective and sustainable programme was group programme 2 (to be found in Appendix A). It consists of techniques of exercise, relaxation and information on nutrition and diet. It should be noted the many participants in this group had problems with work, both emanating from work or because of loss of work.

The other successful stress management programme was programme 1 (see Appendix A) which was the same a programme 2 but included some detail on the cognitive-behavioural control of stress. The programme which used group work which includes creative work such as knitting and crocheting, woodwork and small building projects, was also very successful.

> *Undoubtedly, one of the ways that people in impoverished circumstances can change their lives is by learning to manage their stress within the situation in which they live. This is something that is possible. Their impoverished situation is not likely to change for a long time*

(Crouch 2008, p. 84).

(The reader is asked to go to Appendix A which gives details of stress management programmes which can be used in the community.)

Case Study: Community Stress Management with Active Geriatrics – 'The stress of aging'

An occupational therapist working in the urban community in South Africa ran frequent seminars/workshops with groups of elderly men and women (geriatrics over the age of 70) in a retirement village. The seminars were entitled 'Life stress in the elderly'. The seminar took place once a week for four weeks and was repeated at intervals throughout the year.

These were large groups of about 15–20 participants who were often split up into smaller groups during the group process. The stress management programme was an adapted version of **Appendix A Stress Management Programme P3.**

The occupational therapist tried where possible to make sure that each participant was functioning at the level of Active Participation (Van der Reyden and Sherwood, VdTMoCA 2019) or above but because they voluntarily came to the group it was difficult to control. Psycho-geriatrics are difficult to control in this type of group and takes up the groups precious time.

The occupational therapist was not always able to turn people away.

The aims of the groups were:

- To create an awareness of stress in the elderly and what it is caused by.
- Internal and external pressures and demands on the elderly caused by the environment. These are physical barriers and changes, such as getting in and out of cars, the bath, chairs, etc. due to physical limitations, trying to keep up with technology such as cell phones, computers and electronic equipment. Lack of hearing and poor eyesight contributes greatly to these demands. Pressures and demands by the family were often discussed such as being forced into a retirement home and lack of finances.
- What stress actually does to the body and mind?
- How the elderly tend to create their own stress due to frustration, trying to do what they did in the 'old days', losing their temper, being irritable with others and 'overdoing things'.
- To learn how to recognise and cope with stress in the best possible way. How to balance one's lifestyle, change how things are accomplished and adapt to being older without causing unhappiness, in other words how to control stress.

Very simple seated-warm ups were used at the beginning of each group such as: shaking hands with the person next to you and introducing yourself, saying a sentence such as 'I am Joan and I am nervous today. Who are you?' The next person responds in the same way. This can be varied by saying what interests you or stating your favourite pudding.

Group members were asked to bring a scarf with them and to tell the group what the scarf reminded them of.

Throwing a ball of string around the group, holding onto the end so a web is created, is always popular.

Filling a balloon with rice, asking everyone who can, to stand and punch the balloon around. Always be careful of group members falling.

Actually beginning the stress management session by asking group members to turn to the person next to them and state what stresses them most. Later this can be shared by the group.

These warm-ups were very popular and greatly enjoyed.

When the warm-up was complete the group members were ready to work on their stress and the real group process began. The occupational group therapist used a democratic approach giving every member time to contribute and be acknowledged by the group. There was no co-therapist and the participants were not asked to lead the group at any time.

At the end of the seminar which took place once a week for four weeks, members were asked to write down what they had experienced. They were extremely reluctant to end off the groups. They thoroughly enjoyed the social contact and feedback about their knowledge of controlling their stress was positive.

CHAPTER 14

Practical Creative Activity-Based Group Work in Various Clinical Settings, Including Hospital-Based Group Work with Acutely Ill Mentally Ill Clients

There has always been a debate in the profession of occupational therapy as to whether practical activity-based groups such as craft/creative, discussion, current affairs (newspaper), home-management, childcare, etc. are occupational group therapy (please refer to Section 1.2). Research on occupational group therapy is quite often centred around the use of activities and creative pursuits in occupational group work. Kramer, Nelson and Duncombe as far back as 1984 studied the outcome of the types of activities with chronic psychiatric patients and Duncombe and Howe (1985) did a

Occupational Group Therapy, First Edition. Rosemary Crouch.
© 2021 John Wiley & Sons Ltd. Published 2021 by John Wiley & Sons Ltd.

survey of group work in occupational therapy also in 1985 which consisted of a survey into activities that occupational therapists use in groups.

Authors such as Jennifer Creek and Linda Finlay strongly support creative activity-based group work and the author's experience with Catherine Shorten, Occupational Therapy Technician (OTT) over 19 years in an outpatient setting with mentally ill clients has been extremely positive (see description below).

Task accomplishment is not the only purpose of the group (Shorten and Crouch, in Crouch and Alers 2014) but hopefully the means by which purpose is realised. It is seen as the catalytic agent which elicits behaviour and interaction, brings into focus both the functional capacities and limitations, facilitates collaboration in working through problems and provides a concrete reality factor against which to measure learning and achievement (p. 27). The given task of the activity group may serve the needs of the members in different ways. Creek states that 'Creative activities require the individual to incorporate something of himself into the production of an idea or end product, for example a poem or a piece of embroidery' (Finlay in Creek 2002, p. 265). She also states that 'When someone is facing difficulties due to illness or disability, a capacity for thinking and acting creatively will influence the way in which problems are approached and will enhance the ability to find solutions' (p. 267). In some cases, group members may feel more comfortable working on a task than on interpersonal relationships. These members of the group identify themselves with the group through the involvement with the task activity and need the opportunity to learn how to solve specific problems through participation in joint activity and feel more comfortable working on the task Mosey (1986, p. 28) six major types of activity groups.

The group is mostly dependent on the leader to select and structure the task, particularly in the early stages. The leader is also responsible for creating a group climate that facilitates the interaction of the members, support and tends to the needs of individuals and the group as a whole. He or she must also select appropriate activities or help the group to do so and structure the activities which are suitable at the group member's level of creative ability (Van der Reyden and Sherwood, VdTMoCA 2019). He/she must also guide the learning of interpersonal and task skills which are part of carrying out the activity.

Today the scenario has changed in some countries and occupational therapists have the valued assistance of trained occupational therapy assistants or technicians – OTTs and OTAs as they are known in South Africa. The use of creative activities in groups is greatly enhanced by the expert assistant of these mid-level health workers in many clinical situations.

An Example of a Community-Based Occupational Group Therapy Practice Using Creative Activity Groups

A group practice was opened in Johannesburg in 1993, in answer to a need for a therapeutic support and holding venue for persons discharged from intensive psychiatric hospital care. There is still to this day, a serious need for the continuation of psychiatric care for a considerable portion of the community for this kind of aftercare so that psychiatric treatment can continue into the community and clients can be successfully treated and returned to their occupations. The occupations could be housekeeper and mother, mother/ father and provider in the work community, artist or sportsman, grandmother looking after grandchildren, just a person living on their own, etc.

The practice was run by a registered occupational therapist who employed a registered occupational therapy technician (OTT). The practice was situated in an urban environment as a separate part of a house with four large rooms, an independent entrance and was accessible by bus, taxi or private transport and clients could walk to the practice. There was a garden and a relaxed and inviting setup. Tea and coffee were provided on the verandah and toilet facilities were in the building.

The practice was opened as a request from both public sector and private psychiatric practices in Johannesburg. These practices consisted of psychiatrists and clinical psychologists. The majority

(*continued*)

(continued)

of referrals came from these practices but occasionally referrals were received from social workers, psychiatric nurses and physiotherapists. Of course referrals were also received from community members who wished their charges to receive occupational therapy and they were referred to the psychiatric practices or taken on board with recommendations from professionals working in the mental health field. Medical insurance as well as public sector charges were employed according to the rules abiding at the time.

All interventions were occupational group therapy. However all clients were assessed by the occupational therapist individually, either in hospital before they were discharged or at the practice before therapy commenced. Assessment by the COPM or the VdTMoCA and only patients who were on the level of passive participation and above were accepted into the group. A maximum of 12 patients at a time was accommodated. The ratio of male/female was usually eight females to four males but it varied. Clients were confined to over the age of 18 and an age limit of 70 was imposed. Age is a rule of thumb and it would depend on the level of functioning of the client whether they were accepted for the group or not.

The programme:

The Morning Creative Activity Group

Despite publications to the contrary, the author and authors such as Jennifer Creek (Finlay in Creek 2002) stand firm as to the therapeutic value of a creative activity group. The group gave community clients purpose. They had to get dressed, groom themselves and get themselves to the practice. They were in the company of others with similar problems with which they could relate, learnt to socialise and make friends, often for the first time. They took home useful, acceptable articles for which their families and friends were delighted. The occupational therapist and OTT had time to assess the performance and pathology of their clients and were able to feedback information to the referring doctors on a regular basis. People recovered to their maximum capability and also learnt to live with a mental illness.

A maximum of 10 clients were in the group which obviously changed over time as people recovered and new clients came in. The principle diagnoses were depressive and anxiety disorders, bipolar disorders, substance-use disorders, Asperger's syndrome and schizophrenia. Comorbid conditions included traumatic brain injury, cerebral vascular accident, blindness and on two occasions Huntington's chorea. All clients were formally assessed before commencing in the group and assessed at regular intervals throughout their treatment period. The OTT contributed to this assessment.

The group took place for four hours three times a week with a break for tea in the middle. When clients arrived they took part in a 20 minute exercise, stretching and breathing session outside to start the day off.

The OTT had prepared the activities for the clients and before they started, and the occupational therapist had a brief session to see how everyone was coping and to introduce new clients.

Creative activates used: (Figures 14.1–14.3)

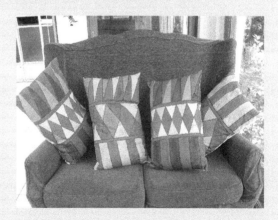

FIGURE 14.1 Fabric painting. One of the most successful activities as it is easy to accomplish. *Source*: Catherine Shorten.

(continued)

(continued)

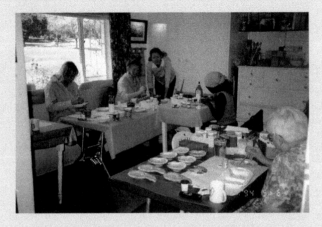

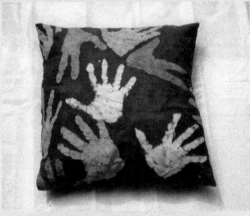

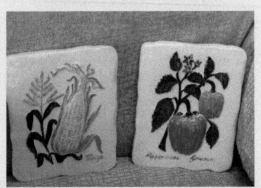

FIGURE 14.2 An occupational therapy technician (OTT) working with a group of clients in the activity group. A cushion made by using a batik technique and ceramics are a very suitable activity for psychiatric clients. *Source*: Catherine Shorten.

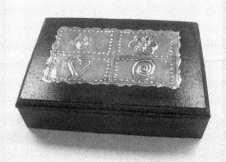

FIGURE 14.3 A varnished box with a pewter modeled top. This is a favourite activity with higher functioning clients. *Source*: Catherine Shorten.

Découpage.
Fabric painting and stencilling.
Pewter work.
Papiere maché.
Ceramics.
Rug-making and embroidery.
Cooking, candle-making, flower-arranging and marbelling (usually done as a workshop where everyone did the same activity).
Wood-burning.
Bead-making.

Some of the gentlemen and the occasional female group member, who was not interested in art activities, undertook puzzles and written activates. Clients were also encouraged to bring their own activities if they so wished and on a number of occasions clients who were artists brought their own canvasses and materials and painted.

The standard of activity was kept high so that clients could be proud and satisfied by what they had achieved and learnt.

Follow-up assessment using the Law et al. (1994) confirmed high levels of satisfaction and development in occupational performance.

14.1   HOSPITAL-BASED GROUP WORK WITH ACUTELY DISTURBED MENTALLY ILL CLIENTS

The use of therapeutic groups remains a core part of occupational therapy practice in the acute mental health setting.

(Cole 2014 in Creek and Lougher).

Group work in this situation, however, has a different dimension because of the short stay of patients in these hospitals in most parts of the world. Chantal Christopher in 2019 stated that 'Group therapy in South African public and private institutions have been influenced by context, particularly in terms of length of stay, the cost implications as approved by the medical aid, as well as the composition and purview of the multidisciplinary team' (p. 9). This implies that there is not time to develop a truly cohesive group and therefore the dynamics are different. For this reason the occupational group therapist has to adapt the group so that the maximum potential from intervention can be realised 'the creation of a supportive group environment with a strong focus on applying skills consistently'. 'therapy should address systemic issues that foster, create or exacerbate mental health conditions' (Christopher 2019, p. 9). This is not easy.

As pointed out by Shorten and Crouch (in Crouch and Alers 2014) the occupational therapy programme is an integral part of the acute stage of mental illness and group work is usually part of the programme. Crouch in 1983 proved that group work in an acute setting was a very effective procedure in which to assess an acutely ill person. Assessment is a vitally important procedure in this setting as the future treatment of all disciplines in the multidisciplinary team is based on this short hospital stay. So many vitally important future aspects of the patient's life depend on it.

'In the acute psychiatric setting, mostly activity-orientated groups are presented as disturbed patients are not suitable for more in-depth and emotionally centred groups' (Shorten and Crouch in Crouch and Alers 2014, p. 122). Occupational therapists are the most highly trained professionals worldwide who provide this essential type of intervention.

It is extremely important for an occupational therapist or occupational therapy technician (OTT) to remain very focussed and confident in the work that they do as there is a tendency to pass their expertise off as 'keeping the patients occupied'. This is indeed not the case and occupational therapists provide a unique service. Not only are they highly trained in this area of practice but they are the only professionals who provide this service. The reader must be reminded that it is therapy!

Typical groups are discussion/education, simple food preparation such as sandwiches and pizzas, creative activities such as crafts, stencilling and fabric painting, lifestyle management groups including leisure activities, budgeting and child and home-management (where appropriate). It must be remembered that today this type of preparation for a seriously mentally ill patient is urgent and essential if they are going to be able to cope after a brief period of treatment and a quick discharge. 'Discharge planning has to begin at the time of admission' (Shorten and Crouch 2014, p. 122).

Discharge must be prepared. In some countries backup and community services are better than others. It is the very best scenario and clients are very privileged if they have an occupational therapy programme in the community to continue with rehabilitation. Group work is the most economic and preferred method of intervention. Other groups are also available from other disciplines such as social work. In a country like Australia, very excellent half-way facilities with day programmes are provided in the communities and sophisticated group programmes such an assertiveness training and stress management take place. They are implemented by community services and led by some professionals such as occupational therapists and community leaders (see Chapter 12).

Lloyd and Williams (2010) stated that 'In such situations occupational therapists are required to engage in a full range of services, from assessment to active treatment, with a focus on assisting service users to engage in meaningful occupational roles both during and after their admission' (p. 437).

CHAPTER 15

Maximising Occupational Group Therapy in Physical Rehabilitation

Occupational group therapy with the physically injured and disabled and with persons with chronic diseases has been very slow to develop in South Africa, yet it is so very important. Support groups, however for people in this field, are active such as the rheumatoid arthritis support group, the traumatic brain injury group, the motor neuron group and the stroke society. Also support groups for the parents and carers of people with physical disability etc. are commonly found in the community and be it an occupational therapist or trained lay person, it is hoped that this book may be of assistance. Skill is required for the leaders of these groups.

An excellent article appeared in the Occupational Therapy International Journal (OTI) in 2011 (Gulati et al. 2011). The subject is adolescent empowerment and it demonstrates and proves that group-centred occupations empower adolescents with disabilities. The power of using group work is demonstrated in this research. It stresses group participation, group demonstration and group recognition.

Also to be found in OTI in 1997 is an article on a work-oriented occupational therapy programme for individuals with physical disabilities by Jang et al. The outcome of this research states that: 'the identified strengths of the programme are: it was an integral part of the rehabilitation process; the programme helped clients to confront their disability and psychosocial dysfunction directly through the individual or group discussion and therapy' (1997, p. 304). It is expected of all occupational therapists working in the so-called 'physical field', e.g. in a spinal unit, to deal with all aspects of rehabilitation. The importance attached to the mental rehabilitation of newly physically disabled patients/clients has grown enormously over the last few years. In many instances, the causes of the disability are either trauma or violence related.

In August 2004, Elma Burger, Deputy Director of Health Therapy at the time in the Gauteng Department of Health stated that 'Group therapy forms an integral part of the occupational therapists' intervention in the physical field and is regarded as essential'.

The possibilities of the use of the therapeutic group process in the physical field are vast and research is urgently needed at a clinical level on every day interventions. The types of occupational group therapy could be as follows:

- Groups to facilitate psychosocial adjustment to a disability or illness.
- Educational groups.
- Skills training groups such as stress management and assertiveness.
- Team-building groups.
- Group empowerment.

The aims of using occupational group therapy in the physical field can be suggested as:

- Developing a milieu where clients/patients feel accepted and belong.

- Facilitation of the sharing of ideas, emotions and problems.
- Influence as to the changing of attitudes.
- Development of identity, confidence and self-esteem.
- Stimulation of motivation to carry out a task.
- Conflict resolution.
- Effective resource utilisation and cost-effectiveness.
- Education and discussion as to coping with sexual difficulties, handling children, mobility issues, dealing with attitudes of the community including issues of prejudice, practical issues such as transportation, reaching items on a grocery store shelf, asking others to help, etc. are all issues and can be very effectively dealt with in a close group.

Types of physical conditions or illnesses where occupational group therapy could be utilised are many but certain conditions such as spinal injuries, amputations, arthritis, physical conditions of the elderly and normal children with physical disabilities come to mind.

There is no difference in the technique of leading a group for the occupational therapist. All the above chapters apply. Allowances will have to be made to accommodate the physical condition.

Appendix A: Community Stress Management Manual

INTRODUCTION

Stress Management Programmes

This manual consists of the outcomes of three years of research in the rural community of the Gazankulu area of Limpopo Province in South Africa.

The research was aimed at the evaluation and development of effective stress management programmes in an underprivileged, rural environment where the stress of the community members is related to both psychosocial and environmental factors.

The Stress Management Programmes

Three stress management programmes will be presented in this manual for use by occupational therapists in the community and if appropriate in other clinical settings.

The most successful programme was Programme 1 that deals mostly with the health of the body. The programme consists of exercise, relaxation and nutrition. It will be presented first in this manual. Please note that colloquial language is used.

Occupational Group Therapy, First Edition. Rosemary Crouch.
© 2021 John Wiley & Sons Ltd. Published 2021 by John Wiley & Sons Ltd.

Programmes P2, a combination of mind and body programme, and Programme P3, dealing only with the mind, are also presented in the manual and are recommended for use as an alternative or perhaps as a change for participants. All three programmes proved to be effective in the alleviation of stress in a community setting.

The Questionnaires – Assessments of Stress

Two questionnaires were used in the research and are presented in this manual for use by the person presenting the stress management programmes.

You will find the questionnaires at the end of the manual and you are welcome to photocopy them for use. Please note that if you decide to change the questionnaires in any way you must state on the questionnaire that it is adapted from the author's original research.

STRESS MANAGEMENT NOTES

These notes are to be used by the person presenting the stress management programme.

Section 1: Introduction to Stress Management

Most people in the community hear the word stress quite often. Few people really understand what it really means and how it can affect you. They often do not understand that a little stress can be good for you and that too much stress can be bad for you.

Stress management is learning how to control too much stress and help it go away. This is very important for the stressed people in our communities.

It is hoped that this programme that will be introduced to you will teach you ways to try and handle stress in your lives. It is important that ways to cope with stress become part of your lives. Just hearing about it is not enough. You need to practise it and change some things to make life easier. It is always possible to change our lives, even when people live in difficult conditions.

Section 2: What Is Stress?

Stress is the way the body and the mind react to pressures and demands made on them. For example, when the children are always asking for money and we do not have any to give them, we get a headache or a pain in the chest, or we get very tired. *(Use more examples here, from the community.)*

Stress is not the same for every person. One person can be much stressed because the porridge burnt, or the mielies are not as good as last year, and another person would not care. *(Use your own examples here.)*

We also know that one person can cope with a lot more stress than another person can. Some people are calm and easygoing and other people are stressed at the smallest thing.

It is important to know that not all stress is bad. We have to have some stress to keep us going – getting up in the morning, getting the children to school, going to see our parents, ploughing the fields. This makes us interested in life, but when stress becomes too much it affects us in a bad way.

Section 3: What Causes Stress?

There are many reasons why people are stressed.

N.B. It is important to ask your group members what it is that makes them stressed.

Examples of reasons why people get stressed could be:

- Frustration with unemployment.
- Frustration and pressure from family and friends.
- Pressure from work.
- In poor living conditions, e.g. poor housing, no money.
- When other people expect us to do things that we do not have time for.
- Doing too much for everyone and not leaving time for ourselves.
- Anxiety and fear.
- Conflict. Argument with the family, or neighbours or friends at work.

- Changes in the family and the environment, like moving to a different place.
- Drinking and drug-taking in the family and amongst friends.
- Poverty issues.
- Lack of education.

Section 4: When Does Stress Become a Problem?

Stress becomes a problem when we cannot get rid of it and it stays with us all the time. Then the symptoms of stress begin to show such as:

- Becoming irritable and irritated.
- Failing to control ourselves.
- Feeling very worried.
- Thinking about problems.
- Keeping away from people. Preferring to be alone.
- Feeling that life is too difficult for us.
- Feeling anxious.
- Feeling tired and sleepy.
- Saying I am not coping, not handling life, not managing.
- Having headaches, pains, aches, etc.

Some illnesses, such as problems with the heart, high blood pressure and difficulty with breathing, can be caused by stress.

It is important to talk about people's symptoms of stress here, but be careful not to go on too long with everyone's general ailments!

Tell the group that if some of these things are a problem, then stress management is important for them.

Section 5: How Do We Make Stress for Ourselves?

It is very important to learn that for some of the time we make our own stress, even if we have a lot of stress coming from outside of ourselves. Stress is not only caused by actual situations but is often caused by imagined or anticipated ones. People's attitudes also cause them stress.

It is hard to believe this, so here is a list of ways we make our own stress.

Physical Ways of Making Our Own Stress

Some people eat and drink a lot of bad food when they are stressed – food with lots of fat and salt and sugar in it, e.g. vet-koek, chips, sweets, cool drinks. These are expensive and have no good in them.

- Some people do not eat at all when they are stressed, even when food is available. The body becomes very tired and sick when it does not have the right kind of food in it. It then becomes more stressed.
- Some people drink a lot of alcohol when they are stressed. This makes the body and mind even more stressed. When under the influence of alcohol people do things that are unacceptable to others (and to themselves) and the guilt of this the next day makes him/her even more stressed.
- Some people spend a lot of time just sitting and doing nothing. This is very bad because the body slows down and becomes sluggish. The blood does not flow nicely and the body becomes stressed.
- Some people take a lot of headache powders and tablets when they are stressed. This is very bad for the body because it affects the kidneys and the liver. When people take a lot it actually causes the headache! This makes the body even more stressed and also costs a lot of money, which makes us even more stressed.

There may be other things participants talk about that can be added to this list.

Cognitive (Our Thoughts) Ways of Making Our Own Stress

- Some people worry all the time about the things they have to do and they worry a lot about other people's problems too.
- Some people cannot say 'no' to other people, such as family members, our children and parents. This is also a traditional custom. We tend to listen to everyone else's problems, take on

work for other people, until we are exhausted. Then there is not enough time for ourselves and to run our own lives.

- Some people often put off things until tomorrow, and then worry about it all the time. The reason they put things off is because it is something they do not want to do, or they are scared to do it or are too stressed to do it today. This is called procrastination and causes ourselves, and other people, lots of stress.

- Many people have negative thoughts, much of the time, particularly people who are suffering from poverty and illness. They never believe anything will go well. In fact they prefer to think that everything will be bad. It is easier. Even some people who are in better circumstances think like this. This is a very severe stressor that we can learn to keep under control.

- Some people spend the little money they have, on the wrong things. Their thoughts play havoc with them! They think they are rich and buy expensive clothes or alcohol, instead of food for the family. This is a severe stressor.

- Guilt about something we have done or said causes a lot of stress. Sometimes we never ever tell anyone about it and we keep this guilt in our minds for a long time.

There may be many other things participants talk about that can be added to this list.

Section 6: Learning to Manage Stress: How to Cope with Your Stress

Physical Ways of Managing Stress

Exercise

People who carry out physical exercise regularly through their everyday work or by sport will keep their stress levels low. Good exercise that needs lots of energy is a distraction from bad thoughts, and provides a break from the stressful environment. Uncomfortable feelings will go away temporarily when you exercise and then they may permanently disappear.

Regular exercise is very important. Walk smartly and briskly, instead of dragging your feet. Walking and running/jogging are the best exercise and they do not cost any money.

Soccer and sports such as basketball are good exercises for men. Sweeping out a room, digging in the garden and ploughing are very healthy exercises and should not be just seen as hard work. Hard work makes people healthy. This is also exercise that is productive! Please note that attitudes to the above types of exercise are cultural and difficult to change.

Try to encourage your participants to do exercises every day.

Relaxation

Relaxation techniques are something that are unfamiliar to a lot of people in the community. Nevertheless it is the quickest way of getting rid of stress, and, although unfamiliar, is going to be taught in some of the stress management programmes. It has been proved to improve health and well-being. Through relaxation the harmful effect of stress can be minimised.

You will have to find a quiet place, sit down and allow yourself at least 10 minutes to yourself. This is difficult but it does not harm to tell the children and other members of the family to let you have 10 minutes of quietness to yourself. You deserve it! Do not feel guilty about it!

After you have discussed relaxation it is important to discuss sleep.

It is important to get at least six hours of sleep. If you are not sleeping well or wake up in the middle of the night or early morning worrying about problems, you must try the relaxation you have been taught and you will soon go back to sleep.

If you have warm milk available, drink some before you go to sleep and you will sleep well.

Nutrition: Good Eating Habits

In this section we learn how to balance stress with a healthy diet. You will be introduced to foods that are good and not good for you. You can eat correctly to get rid of your stress. This is very important!

Do not spend the little money that you have on rubbish. Non-nutritious rubbish includes:

- Cold drinks in tins or bottles. Diet cold drinks are particularly bad for you, as they are full of chemicals, which make your body full of water. There is no goodness for you in these drinks.
- Packets of chips that are full of salt and fat and are very expensive.
- White bread.
- Fatty foods such as fat cakes, fatty meat, fried foods.

Try to eat fruit as often as possible. In many rural areas fruits such as mangos, bananas and paw-paws (papayas) are growing in every village. They are the very best food to eat.

Also try to eat raw or cooked vegetables as often as possible. Try to grow your own.

Some local trees have nuts on them including the Maroela fruit which has kernels in the middle of the fruit. They are very good for stress! Try to get as many as you can from all of the Maroela and other trees near you, during the season. Nuts, including groundnuts, of all kinds are very good food.

Cow's and goat's milk and cheese are good for you, if you can get them.

Use brown or whole-wheat bread only. White bread has very little good food in it.

Try to use cereals and porridge such as mielie-meal, maltabella and oats at the beginning of the day to give you energy, to keep your stress level low and to give you good nutrition.

Cut down on using too much salt, especially if you have high blood pressure. In this case you should not use salt at all. It can cause you to have a stroke. *(Explain what this means.)*

Drink lots of fresh water. Coffee and chocolate contain caffeine and this is why we like them so much. They make us feel good but they also increase the tension in the body. Tea has much less caffeine and is better for you – and cheaper!

Try to use what food you have to the best advantage for your health and your stress. If your health is improved so will your stress! Stop spending money on rubbish foods such as chips and coke. Use the fruits available locally, the spinach growing in your garden, the tomatoes and onions, and the sour and fresh milk available.

Make sure that you start the day with the little food you have available. This will help a lot in keeping your stress levels low. It is very important for children, wherever possible, to go to school with something in their tummies. They will not be able to concentrate on their schoolwork unless they have eaten a fruit or porridge. Do not give them your precious money to buy chips and cold-drinks! Try to change this habit.

When you are eating you should be relaxing at the same time, so that the body can absorb the vitamins and minerals. Take time to digest your food; 20 minutes or half-an-hour is enough.

In many communities, however, eating is a relaxing group event.

Learning to Think Differently to Help Manage Our Stress

Change Your Attitude and Learning to Think Positively

A very important part of this stress management programme is to provide group members with self-help skills which will improve their self-esteem and control and teach them how to take more responsibility for their own well-being. To do this it is important to try and change attitudes.

It is difficult to change attitudes, particularly when people are trying very hard to survive and there is not enough money or food. However, it can be done, by teaching people about positive thinking (e.g. it is going to be a good day today. The sun is shining and I am going to make the best of what I have). We all know that some of the poorest people have a big smile on their face and share the little they have with everyone. These are the positive people who are much less stressed than the negative people.

Negative people always dwell on the problems and make everyone else miserable (e.g. today is going to be another terrible day. Nobody brings me food, the children are naughty and I just will not be able to manage any of it.).

Although we can understand why people think negatively, it is very important to know that if every day you tell yourself that everything is going to go wrong, you can be sure that it will. You actually make it that way by your thinking. At the same time you will be making yourself stressed and everyone else around you. This is one of the reasons why people living in poverty sometimes never learn to rise above it. Negative thoughts stress you and pull you down.

Use some examples of negative thoughts here, from your community, e.g. it is no good planting crops because it is never going to rain, or I am not going to the burial society group today because people will not want to see me.

Even in the poorest circumstances, something positive can be found.

Take some time on this subject. It is very important.

Practise some positive thoughts such as:

- Today is going to be a good day.
- The children are going to do well at school this term.
- I am going to see a friend to make him/her happy again.
- I am going to make the very best of what I have got.

Once a person's attitude becomes positive, then the action following is more likely to be positive too. Until this attitude is changed it is often not possible to move ahead.

Talk About the Things That Worry You

Find a good friend or counsellor that you can trust. Get the problem off your mind and you will reduce your stress.

This we know is not the cultural custom of people in some communities and must be introduced gently.

If you can find a friend who you can really trust, it helps a lot to be able to talk about your problems. Be very careful of people who talk behind your back and cause you more stress.

It is not a good idea to bottle up your problems inside your body. Do not always keep them to yourself. When you talk about your problems, you often think about them differently.

Often a religious leader, or the community rehabilitation/field worker, occupational therapy technician, the social worker or nurse in the local clinic, can be a good person to talk to confidentially.

Let it out!

The Mental Shrug

When we are faced with a situation that is unable to be changed and when we come across small things that do not matter we often become very stressed unnecessarily. We need to learn to shrug the problem off. Lift up the shoulders, make a sigh and make a decision in your head – 'who cares'. Of course this does not mean that we can do this if there is a serious or important problem!

When you have described this and given them an example of something that does not really matter, get the participants to practice the mental shrug. It is always very popular!

Good Time Management

Be kind to yourself and give yourself time. Do something you enjoy every day because you are a very important person. Learn a new skill.

Tell the children to go outside and play while you relax for a while. Look after yourself and your health. What will the family do if you get sick? Think about it! Change your attitude towards yourself.

Do not put off things that can be easily done today. Finish them and get rid of them because they will continue to stress you.

Make a special time to do things that you do not like doing. Do them, finish them and then relax.

Do not take on too much from other people. Learn to say 'no' nicely, to people who put pressure on you, particularly people who are always trying to get you to solve their problems. Try not to feel guilty about this. Tell them the reason that you cannot do it, so that they understand.

This is another cultural issue and will have to be introduced in a sensitive way. It is nevertheless very important, as many people in rural communities are overburdened.

Learn to stand up for your rights. You might feel bad at first but you will find that it will relieve you of your stress. There are only so many hours in a day and thinking about how they should be used will help you with your stress.

Learn to try to get to places on time. Lateness causes you and everyone else stress. Just start your planning a little earlier, leaving time for problems like a taxi being late or a long way to walk.

Section 7: Bad Ways of Getting Rid of Stress

Unfortunately we all try sometimes to get rid of our stress by hurting other people or ourselves. These are considered bad ways of coping with stress.

These are some of the ways we do this:

- Being cross and angry with people, usually the people we love best. We tend to take out our stress on the children and other family members this way. It actually increases the stress for everyone.
- Withdrawing from other people and wanting to always be on our own.
- Taking alcohol or lots of headache powders to help cope with the stress.
- Becoming very involved with activities away from the home so that you can avoid the problems and stress at home. These may be church activities or work for the community that take up so much of your time that you do not have time for important things at home.
- When food is available, some people try to get rid of their stress by eating too much and becoming very fat. Eating a lot makes you feel better for a short time only. When you become very fat you become very stressed at the same time.

Section 8: Learning to Control Your Stress

Stress management is something that needs to be worked on over a period of time. It is hard to change our habits, but it can be done. This will lead to a much better quality of life and you will be happier.

Stress management should not cost us any money. We must learn to use what we have available in the environment to the best possible advantage. We must also learn not to make our own stress!

Please start making changes now and you will notice that you feel much better about yourself. You will feel healthier and the people around you will notice the difference.

A RELAXATION TECHNIQUE

There are many different techniques of relaxation. This is an example of relaxation, which was tried and tested in the research and found to be acceptable in rural communities.

Firstly make sure that your group members are in a quiet place. Ask children to be quiet, shut the door if possible and close the windows.

Relaxation can be done in the lying or sitting position. In the research the sitting position was used because it is easier to fit more people into a small room.

Ask everyone to sit in a comfortable position. Do not allow crossed legs and ask everyone to keep their head up straight.

Start with everyone moving their shoulders around to get rid of the tension in the shoulders. Do it about four or five times. Ask them to bring their shoulders up to their ears and then drop them. Do this twice.

Ask everyone to shut his or her eyes. If they feel uncomfortable doing this then they can look down but not let the head fall forward.

Start with taking a deep breath through the nose, holding the breath for a short while and then breathing out through the mouth slowly. Repeat this.

Ask everyone to stretch their arms in front of him/her with the hands in a fist and to tighten the muscles hard. At the same time they must take a deep breath again through the nose. Hold the breath and hold the tension. Breathe out and relax the arm muscles. Do this again with the fingers stretched out this time. Relax. Feel how relaxed the arms feel now.

Now tighten the tummy muscles and squeeze the buttocks together. Breathe in as before and hold the tension and the breath. Breathe out and relax. The body is beginning to feel heavy and relaxed.

Now tighten both legs by stretching them out in front. Breathe in at the same time. Hold the tension and the breath. Breathe out and relax. Do this again. Relax.

Bring the shoulders up to your ears and breathe in. Then drop your shoulders and breathe out.

Now breathe normally and smoothly. Try to let the chest relax as you breathe. When you breathe out feel the tension going away from your chest.

Feel the neck relaxing and the face. The forehead feels smooth, the eyes heavy. Let the lower jaw drop slightly with the tongue behind the lower teeth.

The whole of the body feels comfortable and relaxed. Stay like this for two minutes.

Let everyone have a good stretch. Ask them to try and stay relaxed like this for the rest of the day.

Exercises

Clients can stand or sit depending on age or if they are not well. When standing, encourage them to stand up straight, bottom and tummy pulled in.

Stand at a distance from each other.

Start with good breathing. In through the nose and out through the mouth, a few times. Explain how important good breathing is. Good breathing, taking big breaths makes you feel good and lets the blood in your body circulate well. (Beware of people becoming dizzy and falling over, especially the smokers.)

Stand with the legs apart. Put the arms above the head and stretch up to the ceiling first with the right and then the left arm. Let people hang onto a chair if they fall over. Repeat at least six times. Breathe in and out.

Circle the shoulders around at least six times and then the arms. Breathe. Bring your shoulders up to your ears and then drop them. Do it again twice.

Take a big breath and let it out slowly.

Put your right ear on the right shoulder, and then put the left ear on the left shoulder. Repeat three times.

Arms out to the side stretch to the left and then the right at least six times. Breathe.

Arms to the sides stretch down the left leg and then the right at least six times. Breathe.

If the group is fit enough, jog around the room and then on the spot.

End off with the breathing.

You must judge carefully how fit people are. Let them sit down if tired.

SUGGESTIONS FOR STRUCTURING THE STRESS MANAGEMENT PROGRAMMES

The stress management programmes which were used in the research took place over four weeks, one session, once a week for one and a half hours each. This was successful but you may like to change the times to suit you. Do not leave too long between sessions as group members will forget what you have covered in the previous session.

The number of group members will vary but it is nice to have from 10 to 15 group members. These group members should not be under the influence of alcohol or drugs or be mentally ill, showing strange behaviour. However, a person who is stable after a mental illness really needs stress management and would benefit from the programme. These programmes are designed for adults only.

It is often difficult to find a quiet place to carry out the stress management programme, but do your best, particularly if you are using a progamme that has relaxation. The church hall, or a school hall and even a private house would be a good venue. You could ask the sister at the local clinic if you could use a room.

It is very acceptable for the presenter to have notes with him/her and where possible use a black board or paper stuck up on the wall that you can write on, for those group members who are literate, to emphasise important points of your stress management.

At the end of this manual there is a handout which you can have photocopied in colour (expensive) or black and white for group members to take home to remind them of the important aspects of stress management.

If you are going to use the stress questionnaires please take note of the programme notes as it will tell you when to use them.

Enjoy every minute. Your group members will really benefit!

THE STRESS MANAGEMENT PROGRAMMES

Stress Management Programme P1

THIS STRESS MANAGEMENT PROGRAMME CONCENTRATES ON THE PHYSICAL WAY TO RELIEVE STRESS.

PREPARE THE VENUE

Session 1

TO START: Welcome all participants and say a prayer if it is your custom.

The following **SECTIONS** on stress management correspond to the sections in the notes on page 6. It is OK to have the manual with you to assist you.

NOW START THE PROGRAMME.

Section 1: Introduction to stress management.

Section 2: What is stress?

Section 6.1.1: Explanation of why exercise is important.

NEXT: Carry out 10 minutes of exercise (an example is found in the manual on page19)

DISCUSSION AND CLOSURE
Remember to ask them to come back next week.

Session 2

WELCOME AND INTRODUCTION TO THE SESSION
Ask clients if they remember what you did last week.

Section 3: What causes stress?

Section 4: When does stress become a problem?

EXERCISES

Section 6.1.2: Explanation of why relaxation is important

SIMPLE RELAXATION (INSTRUCTIONS ON PAGE 17 OF THE MANUAL)

DISCUSSION AND CLOSURE

Remember to ask them to come back next week.

Session 3

WELCOME AND INTRODUCTION

Ask clients if they remember what you did last week.

Section 5.1 ONLY: How do we make stress for ourselves?

Section 6.1.3: Learning to manage stress with good nutrition and eating habits.

EXERCISES

RELAXATION

DISCUSSION AND CLOSURE

Remember to ask them to come back next week.

Session 4

WELCOME AND INTRODUCTION

Section 7: Bad ways of getting rid of stress

Section 8: Learning to control your stress

EXERCISES

RELAXATION

If you are using the stress Questionnaire 1, this would be a good time to repeat it so that you can see if there has been any improvement in your participants.

Go briefly over the subjects you have been discussing in the whole programme with everyone. Encourage them to continue with the programme on their own or with their families.

THANK ALL PARTICIPANTS IN THE TRADITIONAL MANNER.

CLOSURE.

Stress Management Programme P2

THIS STRESS MANAGEMENT PROGRAMME CONCENTRATES ON THE COMBINATION OF PHYSICAL WAYS AND COGNITIVE-BEHAVIOURAL WAYS OF COPING WITH STRESS.

PREPARE THE VENUE

Session 1

(The following **SECTIONS** on stress management are to be found on page 6 of your manual.)

Section 1: Introduction to stress management.
Section 2: What is stress?
Section 3: What causes stress?
SECTION 6.1.2: Explanation of relaxation and its importance in stress management.
NEXT: Simple relaxation (the notes for relaxation are to be found on page of this manual).

DISCUSSION AND CLOSURE

REMEMBER TO ASK THEM TO COME BACK NEXT WEEK.

Session 2

WELCOME AND INTRODUCTION TO THE SESSION
Ask clients if they remember what you did last week.

SECTION 4: When does stress become a problem?
SECTION 5.2: How do we make stress for ourselves through our thoughts?

SECTION 7: Bad ways of getting rid of stress

RELAXATION

DISCUSSION AND CLOSURE

REMEMBER TO ASK THEM TO COME BACK NEXT WEEK.

Session 3

WELCOME AND INTRODUCTION
  Ask clients if they remember what you did last week.

SECTION 6.2.1: Learning to think differently to help manage our stress. Change our attitudes and learn to think positively.

Section 6.2.2: Talk about things that worry you.

Section 6.2.4: Good time management.

Section 6.1.1: Exercise and its importance.

RELAXATION

DISCUSSION AND CLOSURE

REMEMBER TO ASK THEM TO COME BACK NEXT WEEK.

Session 4

WELCOME AND INTRODUCTION

EXPLAIN THAT THIS WILL BE THE LAST SESSION

Section 6.2.3: The mental shrug.

Section 6.1.3 Nutrition and good eating habits

Section 8: Learning to control your stress

A discussion with the group members about the programme can now take place.

THANK ALL PARTICIPANTS IN THE TRADITIONAL MANNER.

CLOSURE

Stress Management Programme P3

THIS STRESS MANAGEMENT PROGRAMME CONCENTRATES ONLY ON THE COGNITIVE/BEHAVIOURAL WAYS TO COPE WITH STRESS.

PREPARE THE VENUE

Session 1

TO START: Welcome all participants.

Then explain what participants are expected to do as follows:

We will meet for four sessions for one-and-a-half hours every week. Please try very hard to come to all four sessions.

(THE FOLLOWING **SECTIONS** ON STRESS MANAGEMENT ARE TO BE FOUND ON PAGE 6 OF THE MANUAL.)

NOW START THE PROGRAMME.

Section 1: Introduction to stress management.

Section 2: What is stress?

Section 3: What causes stress?

DISCUSSION AND CLOSURE

REMEMBER TO ASK THEM TO COME BACK NEXT WEEK.

Session 2

WELCOME AND INTRODUCTION TO THE SESSION

Ask clients if they remember what you did last week.

Section 4: When does stress become a problem?

Section 5.2: How do we make stress for ourselves through our thoughts?

DISCUSSION AND CLOSURE

Remember to ask them to come back next week.

Session 3

WELCOME AND INTRODUCTION
Ask clients if they remember what you did last week.

Section 6.2.1: Learning to think differently to help manage our stress. Change your attitude and learn to think positively.
Section 6.2.2: Talk about things that worry you and that you keep thinking about.

DISCUSSION AND CLOSURE

REMEMBER TO ASK THEM TO COME BACK NEXT WEEK.

Session 4

WELCOME AND INTRODUCTION

EXPLAIN THAT THIS WILL BE THE LAST SESSION.

Section 6.2.4: Good time management
Section 7: Bad ways of getting rid of stress
Section 8: Learning to control your stress

Have a discussion with the group members about the programme. Go briefly over the subjects you have been discussing in the whole programme with everyone. Encourage them to continue with the programme on their own or with their families.

THANK ALL PARTICIPANTS IN THE TRADITIONAL MANNER.

CLOSURE
The following questionnaires were not psychometrically calibrated but are very useful: The columns should be totalled so that the main stressors of the client can be determined. This questionnaire has been translated into Tsonga (an African language) an occupational therapist working in this area of Africa should contact the author for the translated copy.

QUESTIONNAIRE 1

Stress assessment

Name and Date:

Stress factors

Please make a cross (X) in the section that best describes the client's response to your question.

	Never	Very seldom	Sometimes/ now and then	Don't know	Often/time and again	Very often/ many times	Always
Do you:							
1 Feel that life is too difficult for you							
2 Become irritable/irritated							
3 Fail to control yourself							
4 Feel very worried							
5 Think about problems							
6 Keep away from people/like to be alone							
7 Say: "I'm not coping, not handling life, not managing'							
8 Feel anxious e.g. Tremble, sweat, have dry mouth, sigh							
9 Feel tired and sleepy							
Total:							

Source: Copyright R B Crouch (2008).

QUESTIONNAIRE 2

Psychosocial and Environmental Stressors

Place a tick in either the *yes* or *no* column

A	Do you have problems with your family such as:	Yes	No
1	The recent death of a family member		
2	Health problems in family members		
3	Separation of parents, or you and your partner		
4	Divorce amongst parents or you and your marriage partner		
5	Parents or you and your marriage partner, become strangers to one another		
6	Removal from the home		
7	Remarriage of a parent or yourself or spouse		
8	Sexual or physical abuse in the family		
9	Overprotection by your parents		
10	Neglect of a child		
11	Poor or inadequate discipline in the family		
12	Fighting amongst the children		
13	The birth of a new baby in the family		
14	Heavy drinking amongst family members		
15	No food or little food		
16	Drugs e.g. dagga being used by family members		
B	**Do you have problems in your social environment such as:**		
1	The death or loss of a friend		
2	Poor social support		

3	Living alone		
4	Moving out of your own culture		
5	Discrimination		
6	Retirement from work		
C	**Do you have problems with education such as:**		
1	Illiteracy, not being able to read or write		
2	End of School, learning finished		
D	**Do you have problems with your work such as:**		
1	Told to leave, fired, now unemployed		
2	Feeling that you will lose your job		
3	Trying to cope with more work pressure, and demands. Readjustment		
4	Difficult work conditions		
5	Dissatisfaction with your work		
6	Changes to your work conditions		
7	Difficulty with relationships with bosses		
E	**Do you have problems with housing such as:**		
1	Being homeless		
2	Poor housing		
3	Living in an unsafe environment		
4	Problems with your neighbours or home owner		
F	**Do you have economic, money problems such as:**		
1	No money at all		
2	Not enough money		
3	No support from the welfare		

G	Do you have problems with health-care services such as:		
1	Poor health-care services		
2	No transport to healthcare services		
3	No health-care insurance		
H	Do you have problems with the law such as:		
1	Arrests of your family or friends		
2	Have been to jail yourself		
3	Have been in trouble with police, e.g. given a fine.		
I	Do you have other problems such as:		
1	Seen violence taking place		

Appendix B: Assertiveness

B.1 WHAT IS ASSERTIVENESS?

- 'The ability to relate effectively to the people and situations in our environment.
- A state of being which results from a sense of self-worth and self-confidence.
- A belief in our rights and the rights of others and the ability to communicate effectively.' (Nove 1989, p. PA10)

B.1.1 Lazarus Defines Assertiveness As

- The ability to say NO without feeling guilty (Lazarus 1973).
- The ability to ask for a favour or make requests.
- The ability to express positive and negative feelings.
- The ability to initiate, continue and terminate general conversation.

Self-expression is synonymous with self-assertion – this is the ability to communicate feelings to others, to express friendship and affection, annoyance and anger, joy and pleasure, grief and sadness, and to both give and accept praise and criticism.

Occupational Group Therapy, First Edition. Rosemary Crouch.
© 2021 John Wiley & Sons Ltd. Published 2021 by John Wiley & Sons Ltd.

Assertion is not simply dealing with negative situation but is rather a style which may influence many social interactions. Being assertive does NOT mean being aggressive. When asking the emphasis is on being direct, looking at the other person and making it clear what you want. Eye contact, facial expression and tone of voice are particularly important. Checking out procedures may be a good idea to sound out a person before proceeding, thus minimising the chance of refusal or embarrassment.

There are many situations in which assertive behaviour would be appropriate, and the following examples are just a few of the situations which many people report having difficulty with and which are often included in training programmes.

- Standing up for your rights/not being cheated.
- Making a request/asking someone out.
- Coping with refusal.
- Refusing a request.
- Showing appreciation.
- Making apologies.

B.2   THE CONTINUUM OF ASSERTIVENESS

NON ASSERTION involves violating one's own rights by failing to express honest feelings, thoughts and beliefs, and consequently permitting others to violate us, or expressing our thoughts and feelings in such an apologetic manner that others can easily disregard them.

ASSERTION involves directly standing up for your personal rights and expressing your thoughts, feelings and beliefs in a direct, honest and appropriate way with good timing, which does not violate another person's rights. Thus assertion is 'This is what I think, this is how I feel, and this is how I see the situation'. This is said without dominating, humiliating or degrading the other person.

AGGRESSION involves directly standing up for personal rights and expressing thoughts, feelings and beliefs in a way which is often dishonest, usually inappropriate and always violates the rights of the other person. Aggression is winning by humiliating, degrading or belittling or overpowering the other person so that they become weaker, and less able to defend themselves. An aggressive person usually loses or fails to establish close relationships with others and has to be constantly vigilant against attack from others.

Assertion is a Learned Behaviour, as is Aggression and Non Assertion

B.3   GOALS OF ASSERTION

1. To develop caring, honest and accepting relationships.
2. To get and give respect.
3. To ask for fair play.
4. To leave room for compromise when the needs and rights of two people conflict.
5. To increase self-esteem and self-confidence.

B.4   BENEFITS OF ASSERTIVE BEHAVIOUR

1. To manage our feelings, and not letting them dominate us or force us into submission or attack.
2. To take more risks which allow us to grow and gain self-esteem.
3. To eventually realise a greater ability to deal with conflict openly and fairly, which results in closer, more emotionally satisfying relationships.
4. To give others a chance to know where we stand, and to change their behaviour at their discretion, or to make a compromise for development.
5. To maximise the likelihood of achieving the goal set.
6. To build your own self-esteem, thus increasing your confidence. Accept yourself as you are and be kind to yourself. Identify your behaviour as unacceptable and not yourself as unacceptable.

B.5 DEVELOPING AN ASSERTIVE PHILOSOPHY

1. Assertive behaviour supports the concept of basic human rights.
2. Accepting personal rights does not mean acting in any way you may wish with total disregard for others.
3. Our rights do not negate others rights.
4. Accepting rights brings personal power which also brings responsibility, i.e. we have the responsibility to avoid reckless behaviour and not blame others when we make mistakes. People usually respect and admire those who are responsibly assertive and those who show respect for self and others. Also respect and admiration are shown for those who show courage to stand by their beliefs and deal with conflict fairly and openly.

B.6 DEVELOPING SELF-ESTEEM

'Self-esteem' is a state of mind. It is the way we feel and think about ourselves and others and is measured by the way we act. Self-esteem is made up of learned feelings and positive thoughts that reflect a positive attitude of 'I can do it', versus a pessimistic attitude of 'I can't do it'.

Self-esteem comes from two sources:

1. 'Outside factors such as praise and recognition from others, educational success and valued possessions etc.
2. Inside factors such as the degree of self-acceptance, self-knowledge, awareness of and acceptance of feelings, wants and goals, and the ability to effectively express ourselves in a relationship.

   Balance between these two items is important. For example, people enjoy receiving praise and encouragement from others, but dependence on the "outside" for self-esteem is subject to up and downs which cannot be controlled.

It requires that other people are there when praise is needed. It requires consistent help from relatives, friends, teachers and others. It often means that we have to achieve highly to retain approval and we see ourselves as successful only if others consider us to be so.' (Nove 1989, p. PA11)

Self-esteem therefore has to be developed from the inside. 'If we can learn to meet our own needs for acknowledgement and acceptance, anything which then comes from outside sources becomes a real bonus. People with a solid base of "inside" self esteem tend to feel more comfortable with themselves and others, more in control of their lives and less dependent on others for a sense of well-being.' (Nove 1989, p. PA11)

B.6.1   Being Fair to Self

'How often are people more fair in their attitude to others than to themselves? When someone else does something stupid, it is often easy to offer consolation and positive comments. People rarely think of doing this for themselves, however, and go on blaming themselves for their mistakes.

Focusing on things we do well instead of always noticing the bad things and taking the good for granted is one way of learning to balance the negatives and positives.

Often the things people consider to be faults in themselves can be looked at from a different point-of-view and become positive. For example, those who see themselves as inadequates conversationalists may actually be very good listeners.' (Nove 1989, p. PA14)

B.6.2   Giving to Self

'We have a limited amount of emotional energy which gets depleted in dealing with other adults, children, pressures at work and a host of other tasks. This energy can be replenished by "giving" to self, a practice which varies from person to person. One person like to go for walks alone, another may like to be in a crowd, while others may like to read or sit and daydream or listen to music. Many people grow up believing it is wrong to be "selfish" and instead go to the opposite extreme where they become "self-less", putting their own needs last and denying themselves for others. There is a middle way, a "self thinking" position which meets our own needs (but not at the expense of others) and others' needs (but not at the expense of self).

Giving to self is often a new idea and people may feel guilty taking time for themselves when there are so many demands for service and sharing with others. But giving time and energy to others when our own resources are low results in poor quality giving, often accompanied by irritation and resentment.

We can feel justified, then, in taking time to "give to self", to refill our cup of energy. Where people have limited free time, even a half-hour consciously "given to self" is effective if used regularly and with enjoyment.

Discovering activities which "give to self" can be an adventure. Our lives become so busy that recognising the importance of setting aside special time for ourselves gives us freedom to try new things or take up activities we used to enjoy.

As with all self-confidence tasks, "giving to self" requires practice and conscious effort.' (Nove 1989, p. A14)

B.6.3   Being Responsible for Self

'By taking responsibility for meeting our own needs, building our own self confidence and self-esteem, we can feel much more comfortable about ourselves. We can accept from others without being overly dependent on them. This enables give and take in relationships and a satisfying capacity for sharing and companionship, rather than an unhealthy over-dependence on another to meet our needs for self-confidence and self-esteem.

It becomes a challenge to accept responsibility for one's own thoughts, ideas, words and actions. Taking responsibility in this way encourages others to be responsible for themselves also. We no longer have to take the blame for the mistakes, feelings and behaviour of others.' (Nove 1989, p. A13.)

B.6.4   Being Kind to Self

'Most people think that it is important to be kind to others but forget about being kind to themselves. There are many ways of being kind to self. The ones specified here are:

B.6.4.1   Doing Is Not Being (Labels)

It is very helpful to be able to separate ourselves from our behaviour. While people produce behaviour they do not become that behaviour. Barking like a dog or quacking like a duck does not transform us into a dog or a duck. How often, though, do people fail at a task and call themselves a failure, or do something stupid and call themselves stupid? Trouble begins when labels such as these are accepted as being the whole person. Words are important and if people label themselves or are labeled by others often enough the cumulative effect can be crippling and self-damaging. Becoming more aware of labels ("I am . . ." "You are . . ." etc.) and refusing to accept them, makes it easier to look at what is happening.

Make the distinction between behaviour and self makes it easier to accept ourselves while charging the behaviour. Positive labels can be as destructive as negative ones. The label "coper" can imply an expectation that person is always strong and never weak whichxcan be very uncomfortable when that person wants help.' (Nove 1989, p. A13)

B.6.4.2   Self-talk

People are unfair to themselves when they set unrealistic standards of behaviour and then label themselves as failures when they cannot meet those standards.

These unrealistic standards invariably contain a 'should' (e.g. 'I should be able to cope with any situation'). By modifying the 'should' we take the pressure off having to perform perfectly every time.

'Different people respond differently to the same situation. How they respond can depend on their self-talk, or what they say to themselves about what is happening.

Suppose someone has an accident and needs assistance. One person may rush up and help, saying to himself: "Poor fellow, he needs help". Another may look the other way saying: "Don't get involved". Yet another may become angry, saying to herself: "Stupid idiot, he should be more careful !"

Self-talk goes on constantly as people respond to what is happening around them. It is often unconscious but is always there. Self-talk starts as soon as a child begins to formulate thoughts in order to make sense of the world and continues throughout life. It is an important part of everyday living and happens all the time, whether at a conscious level or not, and is a natural, integrating way of communicating with oneself.

In developing a repertoire of self-talk (silent sentences) people draw on parental messages initially and many people carry these, unaware and unquestioning, into adult life. School and society rules become implanted and messages from any influential people during the developing years – family, other adults or peers – all play a part in determining each person's individual collection of 'silent sentences'. Over the years these become firmly rooted and people act and react according to these well-learned and conditioned responses.' (Nove 1989, p. A16)

Feeling good about yourself is not a luxury; it is an absolute necessity

B.7   SELF-CONFIDENCE

'It is important to note the following:

1. People can build their own self-confidence
2. People can accept themselves as they are.
3. The skills of building self-confidence are:
   a. Being kind to self by changing self-talk and negative thinking
   b. Not trying to always prove oneself by "doing".
4. Self praise.

5. Self-encouragement
6. Being fair to self.
7. Giving to self.
8. Being responsible for self

B.8   SELF CONFIDENCE CAN BE DEVELOPED

Many people grow into adult life believing that self-confidence is primarily dependent on other people's opinion of them. By learning and practising skills such as self-acceptance, people can take responsibility for developing their own self-confidence. It take time, consistent effort and determination to change ineffective patterns of behaviour, but the benefits are obvious and lead to a greater independence, a sense of direction and freedom to establish a fulfilling and creative life.' (Nove 1989, p. A12)

B.9   SENSITIVE AREAS OR 'BUTTONS'

'"Buttons' is a term used to describe sensitive areas an individual may have – areas which, if touched on or pushed, trigger over-reactions to situations or people. These sensitive spots are different for everyone and are usually related to qualities we dislike about ourselves or characteristics we think should be different. To someone who believes that homes should be kept tidy but is a poor housekeeper, comments on the state of tidiness often result in an over-reaction. The feeling may be guilt or resentment and the silent sentences something like: 'I should be a tidy person. Because my house is untidy that means I am less worthwhile than people who keep their houses tidy'.

Learning to recognise our own 'buttons' by acknowledging the over-reaction and the feelings triggered by that particular incident is a very effective way of uncovering the deeply rooted silent sentences behind the button. It is also an essential part of learning to be assertive.

Once the silent sentences are identified we can choose to change them is appropriate.

In a close relationship, mutual awareness of sensitive areas can be helpful in avoiding the upset resulting from pushing buttons."

(Nove 1989, p. B58)

B.10 STEPS TO ASSERTIVENESS

1. Positive assertive communication: This is letting someone know your positive feelings towards them. This also is when you have received a compliment and know how to handle it.
2. Negative assertion: This will be when you admit to an error that you have made.

When choosing to act assertively, the following steps are a useful guideline:

1. Be aware of your feeling and what to do with the feeling.
2. Be aware of your irrational self-talk and challenge any uncomfortable 'should' you find.
3. Be aware of your rights.
4. Decide what to do or say.
5. If you choose to speak, send messages without blame by:
   a. Careful timing.
   b. Using an 'I' statement.
   c. Being congruent (verbal matches nonverbal).
   d. Being specific about other's behaviour.
   e. Acknowledging the other's feelings when appropriate.
6. Keep the 'we' in the relationship and be prepared to negotiate: e.g. 'I can choose to be passive if the risk to the relationship is too great'.

B.11 HANDLING MANIPULATIVE BEHAVIOUR

Manipulative behaviour is when you are manipulated into feeling a way in which you are not comfortable. It is important to recognise and be aware of these situations when manipulative behaviour is being used, e.g. when a person withdraws too readily from the slightest confrontation. When someone has all the answers and is too quick or controlling. When someone is aggressive, unkind or threatening, or extremely critical. When you feel that you are being treated unfairly or unjustly, a clear honest statement of that fact is the single most assertive act that you can make.

1. **Broken record:** Repeating a statement over and over.
2. **Fogging:** Partially agree with the manipulative criticism.
3. **Use of fogging and the broken record:** Partially agree with the manipulative comment but still hold your ground and repeat your stand.
4. **Time out:** Give yourself time to think something over when you are asked an important question for which you are unprepared.

These techniques are sometimes frustrating to the recipient and can possibly lead to alienation. It is best to use open communication, be direct and use protective measures only if necessary.

B.12   IN CONCLUSION

'We are not our feelings. We are not our moods. We are not even our thoughts. The very fact that we can think these things separates us from them and from the animal world. Self-awareness enables us to stand apart and examine even the way we "see" ourselves – our self-paradigm, the most fundamental paradigm of effectiveness. It affects not only our attitudes and behaviors, but also how we see other people. It becomes our map of the basic nature of mankind.' (S. Covey 1994)

B.13   ANGER MANAGEMENT

Disarming anger:
    The goal is to identify with the others feelings until he or she can calm down for a more rational discussion.

B.13.1   Handling Your Own Anger

1. Acknowledge your feelings of anger (use 'I' statements). Owning your anger makes you more in control.
2. Judge the level of your anger. This will indicate to you how you should deal with it.
3. Diagnose the threat (what is the worst that can happen).
4. Share the threat (to diffuse feelings).
5. Physically express feelings (appropriately).
6. Forgive once you have worked through your anger.

B.13.2   Handling Other's Anger Directed Towards You

1. Acknowledge their feelings (to diffuse their anger).
2. Acknowledge your feelings (to be assertive and in control).
3. Use the broken record (to calm them down and get their attention).
4. Renegotiate the relationship.
5. Acknowledge regret (apologise if necessary).

B.14   RECEIVING CRITICISM

1. Anticipate (ask for feedback assertively).
2. Keep calm.
3. Think positively.
4. Listen carefully.
5. Empathise with your critic (do not sympathise).
6. Play for time (when scared/too angry).
7. Share your reaction (acknowledge positive and negative).
8. Give your inner confidence a boost.
9. Work out an action plan.

B.15 GIVING CRITICISM

1. Choose an appropriate time and place (give a warning).
2. Keep calm.
3. Be rational.
4. Acknowledge the positive.
5. Empathise.
6. Be specific (do not generalise), do not label person.
7. Keep to the point.
8. Outline consequences.

B.16 QUESTIONNAIRE 1

B.16.1 Estimate of Self-Concept

This questionnaire is designed to show how you see yourself. It is not a test, so there are no right or wrong answers. Please answer each item as carefully and accurately as you can by placing a number next to each statement.

1. Rarely or never
2. A little of the time
3. Sometimes
4. Often
5. Most or all of the time

1. I feel that people would not like me if they really knew me well. _____
2. I feel that others get along much better than I do. _____
3. I feel that I am an attractive person. _____
4. When I am with other people, I feel they are glad I am with them. _____
5. I feel that people really like to talk to me. _____
6. I feel that I am a competent person. _____

7. I feel that I make a good impression on others. _____
8. I think that I need more self-confidence. _____
9. When I am with strangers, I am very nervous. _____
10. I think that I am a dull person. _____
11. I feel unattractive. _____
12. I feel that others have more fun than I do. _____
13. I feel that I bore people. _____
14. I think my friends find me interesting. _____
15. I think I have a good sense of humour. _____
16. I feel very self-conscious when I am with strangers. _____
17. I feel that if I could be more like other people I would be happy. _____
18. I feel that people have a good time when they are with me. _____
19. I feel embarrassed when I go out. _____
20. I feel I get pushed around more than others. _____
21. I think I am a rather nice person. _____
22. I feel that people really like me very much. _____
23. I feel that I am a likeable person. _____
24. I am afraid I will appear foolish to others. _____
25. My friends think very highly of me. _____

- Reverse the scores for the following items: 3, 4, 5, 6, 7, 14, 15, 18, 21, 22, 23, 25 (e.g. If you entered 2, it becomes 4 and 4 becomes 2, whilst 3 remains the same).
- Total the scores
- 20–30 – your self-concept is very positive.
- 3–50 points – your self-concept is good, problem areas are few.
- 51–80 points – you have a fair self-concept, attention should be given to the problem areas.
- 81–125 points – you have quite a number of problem areas which contributes to a negative self-concept. You can benefit from a skills training course.

Source: From: LIFESKILLS FOR SELF DEVELOPMENT, National Council for Mental Health, October 1986.

RECOMMENDED READING

Covey, R., *The Seven Habits of Highly Effective People*, London: Simon and Schuster, 1994.

B.17   QUESTIONNAIRE 2

B.17.1   Occupational Therapy Assertiveness Assessment

Rate Your Assertiveness Behaviour According to the Following Scale:

0–1 You behave in a passive withdrawn manner
4–6 You behave assertively without difficulty
4–10 You behave aggressively (passive or active aggression).

	Relatives	Friends	Strangers	Authority figures	Sub ordinates	Service people	Groups
Refusing requests							
Handling criticism							
Receiving gifts etc.							
Stating your rights & needs							
Expressing negative feelings							
Giving neg feedback							
Differing from others							
Making requests							
Expressing positive feelings							
Making soc.contact							
Confronting others							
Giving opinions							

Source: From R. B. Crouch (1993).

References

Alers, V.M. (2007) African adventure cards. http://actingthru.org.za/adventurecards.html.

Alers, V.M. and Crouch, R.B. (eds.) (2010). *Occupational Therapy: An African Perspective*. Johannesburg: Sarah Shorten Publishers.

Alers, V. and Smuts, B. (2002). The development and evaluation of an experiential approach to teaching occupational therapy groupwork. *South African Journal of Occupational Therapy* 32 (3): 14–20.

Avnon, E. (1989). Drawing workshops. Po Box 1360, Tivnon 3600 Israel.

Barker, J.A. (1991). The power of vision. www.finestquotes.com. https://www.oxfordreference.com/view/10.1093/acref/9780191826719.001.0001/q-oro-ed4-00011987.

Beynon-Pindar, C. (2017). *Group Work in Occupational Therapy: Generic Versus Specialist Practice*. London: John Wiley and sons.

Blatner, H.A. (1973). *Acting-In Practical Applications of Psychodramatic Methods*. New York: Springer Publishing Company, Inc.

Blatner, A. (1988). *Foundations of Psychodrama: History, Theory and Practice*, 3e. New York: Springer Publishing Company.

Borg, B. and Bruce, M. (1991). *The Group System*. New Jersey: Slack.

Brandes, D. (1982). *Gamesters Handbook Two: More games for teachers and group leaders*. Johannesburg, London: Hutchinson.

Bundey, C., Cullen, J., Denshire, L. et al. (1984). *A Manual about Group Leadership and a Resource for Group Leaders*. Sydney, Australia: NSW: Health Promotion Unit, Program Development Branch, Department of Health.

Burger, E. (2007). Lecture at Baragwanath hospital in Johannesburg (Unpublished lecture).

Casteleijn, D. (2014). Using measurement principles to confirm the levels of creative ability as described in the Vona du Toit model of creative ability. *South African Journal of Occupational Therapy* 44 (1): 14–18.

Casteleijn, D. and Smit, C. (2002). The psychometric properties of the creative participation assessment. *The South African Journal of Occupational Therapy* 32 (1): 6–11.

Christopher, C. (2019). Occupational Therapy Groups as a vehicle to address interpersonal relationship problems: mental care users. *South African Journal of Occupational Therapy* 49 (2) `https://doi.org/10.17159/2310-3833/2019/vol49n2a2`.

Cole, M.B. (2014). Client-centred groups. In: *Creek's Occupational Therapy and Mental Health 2014*, 5e (eds. W. Bryant, J. Fielcharao, J. Banniger, et al.). Oxford: Churchill Livingston/Elsievier.

Covey, S.R. (1994). *The Seven Habits of Highly Effective People*. London: Simon and Shuster.

Creek, J. (2008). Approaches to practice. In: *Occupational Therapy and Mental health*, 4e (eds. J. Creek and L. Lougher), 59–79. Churchill Livingston Elsevier: Edinburgh.

Creek, J. and Bullock, A. (2008). Assessment and outcome measurement. In: *Occupational Therapy and Mental Health*, 4e (eds. J. Creek and L. Lougher), 1–601. Edinburgh: Churchill Livingston.

Creek, J. and Lougher, L. (2008). *Occupational Therapy and Mental Health*, 4e. London: Elsevier.

Crouch, R.B. (1987). A study of the effectiveness of certain occupational therapeutic techniques in the assessment of acutely disturbed adult psychiatric patients. *British Journal of Occupational Therapy* 50 (3): 86–90.

Crouch, R.B. (1992). *Occupational Therapy in Psychiatry and Mental Health*. Johannesburg: Lifecare.

Crouch, R.B. (1993). Assertiveness Training Lecture Notes. University of Witwatersrand (Unpublished).

Crouch, R.B. (2008). A community-based stress management programme for an impoverished population in South Africa. *Occupational*

Therapy International 15 (2): 71–86. Published online 18th February 2008 in Wiley Interscience (www.interscience.wiley.com) DOI: https://doi.org/10.1002/oti.246.

Crouch, R.B. and Alers, V.M. (1997). *Occupational Therapy in Psychiatry and Mental health*, 3. Johannesburg: Maskew Miller Longman.

Crouch, R. and Alers, V.M. (2005). *Occupational Therapy in Psychiatry and Mental Health*, 4e. London: Whurr Publishers.

Crouch, R.B. and Alers, V.M. (2014). *Occupational Therapy in Psychiatry and Mental Health*, 5e. Oxford: Wiley & Blackwell.

Crouch, R. B. and Fouché, L. (2018). *The Concept of Occupational Group Therapy: Rethinking group-work in occupational therapy*. PowerPoint presentation at POTS Symposium, Johannesburg (Unpublished).

Crouch, R. and Mogotsi, M. (2007). Group writing as a work preparation in the vocational rehabilitation of persons with bipolar mood disorders. A research poster presented at the Faculty of Health Sciences Research Day in 2007 at the University of Witwatersrand.

De Beer M and Vorster C (1980) Interactive Groupwork model (IGM) University of Pretoria (Unpublished).

De Witt, P. and Sherwood, W. (2019). Assessment of creative ability. In: *VdTMoCA. The vona du Toit Model of Creative Ability* (eds. D. Van der Reyden, D. Casteleijn, W. Sherwood and P. de Witt). Pretoria: Vona and Marie du Toit Foundation.

Duncombe, L.W. and Howe, C. (1985). Group-work in occupational therapy: a survey of practice. *The American Journal of Occupational Therapy* 39 (3): 163–170.

DuToit, V. (2009). *Patient Volition and Action in Occupational Therapy*, 4e. Pretoria: Pretoria Vona and Marie du Toit Foundation.

Edel, M.-A., Hölter, T., Wassink, K., and Juckle, G. A comparison of mindfulness-based group training and skills group training in adults with ADHD. *J Allen Disorders 2017* 21 (6): 533–539.

Eklund, M. (2006). Therapeutic factors in occupational group therapy identified by patients discharged from a psychiatric day centre and their significant others. *OTI* 14 (3): 200–214.

Eliot, T.S. (1943). *Four Quartets*. New York: Harcourt.

Finlay, L. (2002). Groupwork. In: *Occupational Therapy and Mental Health*, 3e (ed. J. Creek). London: Churchill Livingston.

Fouché, L. (2020). OGIM original lecture notes. Johannesburg.

Gulati, S., Paterson, M., Medves, J., and Cotta Mancini, M. (2011). Adolescent group empowerment: Group-centred occupations to empower adolescents with disabilities in the urban slums of North India. *Occupational Therapy International* 18 (1): 67–84. London, Wiley-Blackwell.

Hagedorn, R. (2000). *Tools for Practice in Occupational Therapy: A Structured Approach to Core Skills and Processes*. Toronto: Harcourt Publishers.

Holmes, P., Karp, M., and Watson, M. (1994). *Psychodrama Since Moreno: Innovations in Theory and Practice*. London: Routledge.

Homans, G.C. (1968). *The Human Group*. London: Routledge and Kegan Paul Ltd.

Howe, M.C. and Schwartzberg, S.L. (1986). *A Functional Approach to Group Work in Occupational Therapy*. London: J.B. Lippincott Co.

Hudgens, K.M. (2002). *Experiential Treatment for PTSD. The Therapeutic Spiral Model*. New York: Springer Publishing Company.

Jang, Y., Mann-Tsong, H., and Li, W. (1997). A work-orientated occupational therapy programme for individuals with physical disabilities. *Occupational Therapy International* 4 (4): 304–316. Whurr Publishers Ltd.

Kielhofner, G. (2002). *A Model of Human Occupation: Theory and Application*, 3e. Baltimore: Lippincott & Wilkins.

Kivlinghan, D.M. (2012). Group Dynamics: Theory, Research and Practice. In: Power in Number (ed. A. Patural). *American Psychological Association* 43 (10): 48.

Law, M., Baptiste, S., Carswell, A. et al. (1994). *The Canadian Occupational Performance Measure*, 2e. Ottawa: CAOT Publications ACE.

Lazarus, A.A. (1973). On assertive behaviour. *Behaviour Therapy* 4: 697–699.

Lesunyane, A. (2010). Psychiatry and mental health in Africa. In: *Occupational Therapy: An African perspective* (eds. V. Alers and R. Crouch). Johannesburg: Sarah Shorten.

Leuner, H. (1969). Guided affective imagery. *A Method of Intensive Psychotherapy* XX111 (1): 4–22.

Lewin, K. (1951) 3-Stage model of change: unfreezing changing and refreezing. Web: Study.Com.

Lloyd, S.R. (1988). *Developing Positive Assertiveness*. California: Crisp Publications Inc.

Lloyd, C. and Maas, F. (1997). Occupational therapy group work in psychiatric settings. *BJOT* 60 (5): 226–230. https://www.researchgatenet/publication/275230621.

Lloyd, C. and Williams, P.L. (2010). Occupational therapy in the modern adult acute mental health setting: a review of current practice. *International Journal of uTherapy and Rehabilitation* 17 (90): 436–442.

Maslow, A. (1962). *Toward a Psychology of Being*. Princeton: Van Nostrand.

Max-Neef, M.A. (1991). *Human Scale Development*. New York and London: The Apex Press.

McLean, H. (1975). An encounter: occupational therapy and psychodrama. *British Journal of Occupational Therapy.* 1975: 163–171.

Mehdizadeh, M., Mehraban, A.H., and Zahedijannasab, R. (2017). Stroke survivors: the effect of group-based occupational therapy on performance and satisfaction of stroke survivors. *Basic Clinical Neuroscience* 8 (1): 69–76.

Moreno, J.L. (1946). *Psychodrama*, vol. 1. New York: Beacon House. (revised 1964). A classic and basic text.

Moreno, J.L. (1953). *Who Shall Survive? Foundations of Sociometry, Group Psychotherapy and Sociodrama*. Beacon: Beacon House.

Moreno, J.L. (1975). *Psychodrama: Action Therapy and Principles of Practise*, vol. 3. New York: Beacon House.

Mosey, A.C. (1973). *Activities Therapy*. New York: Raven Press Publishers.

Mosey, A. (1986). *Psychosocial Components of Occupational Therapy*. New York: Lippincott Williams and Wilkins.

Nove, T. (1989). *A Training Manual on Assertiveness Skills for Community Education and Health*. Sydney State Health Publication, NSW Department of Health.

OTASA, Occupational Therapy Association of South Africa (2014) Scope statement on occupational therapy group-work. www.OTASA.org.za.

Paul, R. (1996). Using standards to intellectual assess student reasoning centre for critical thinking.

Perls, F., Hefferline, R.E., and Goodman, P. (1971). *Gestalt Therapy*. New York: Bantam.

Radnitz, A., Christopher, C., and Gurayah, T. (2019). Occupational therapy groups as a vehicle to address interpersonal relationships problems: mental health care users'. *South African Journal of occupational Therapy* 49 (2): 1–11. Pretoria August 2019.

Ramano, E.M. and de Beer, M. (2017). A comparison of two occupational therapy group programs on the functioning of patients with major depressive disorders. *Minerva Psychiatrica* 58 (3): 125–134.

Ramano, E.M., de Beer, M., Becker, P.J., and Roos, J.L. (2018). Mental health care users with major depressive disorders: Initial outcomes of an occupational therapy group programme. *African Journal for Physical Activity and Health Sciences (AJPHES)* October 2018 (Supplement): 60–71.

Reed, K.L. and Sanderson, S.N. (1983). *Concepts of Occupational Therapy*, 2nde. Baltimore: Williams and Wilkins.

Remocker, A. and Storch, E.T. (1977). *Action Speaks Louder*. Canada: Copyright authors.

Ritchie, J. (1970). *Teaching People to Unwind. A Training Manual on Relaxation and Stress Management Techniques for Community Educators and Health Professionals*. NSW: Health Promotion Unit, Department of Health.

Roberts, M. (2008). Life –skills. In: *Occupational Therapy and Mental Health*, 4e (eds. J. Creek and L. Lougher). London: Elsievier.

Robertson, L. (2012). *Clinical Reasoning in Occupational Therapy Controversies in Practice*. Oxford, UK: Wiley Blackwell.

Rogers, C. (1961). *On Becoming a Person*. Boston: Houghton Mifflin.

Scholl, B.A. and Cervero, R.M. (1993). Clinical reasoning in occupational therapy: an integrative view. *AJOT* 47 (7): 605–610.

Shorten, C. and Crouch, R. (2014). Acute psychiatry and the dynamic short-term intervention of the occupational therapist. In: *Occupational Therapy in Psychiatry and Mental Health*, 5e (eds. R. Crouch and V. Alers). London: Wiley Blackwell.

Shutz, W.C. (1967). *Joy: Expanding Human Awareness*. New York: Grove Press.

Sinclair, K. (2003). A model for the development of clinical reasoning in occupational therapy. Ph.D. thesis. Hong Kong Polytechnic University.

Sinclair, K. (2003). The Sinclair Matrix. In: *Occupational Therapy in Psychiatry and Mental Health*, 5e (eds. R. Crouch and V. Alers). London: Wiley Blackwell.

Townsend, E.A. (1999). Clint-centred Practice. Good Intentions Overruled. *Occupational Therapy Now.* 1 (4): 8–10.

Townsend, E.A. and Polatajko, H.J. (2007). *Enabling Occupation II: Advancing an Occupational Therapy Vision for Health, Well-being, & Justice through Occupation*. Ottawa: CAOT Publications ACE.

Tubbs, S.L. (1978). *A Systems Approach to Small Group Interaction*. New York: Addison-Western Publishing Company.

Tubbs, S.L. and Moss, S. (1981). *Interpersonal Communication*, 2e. New York: Random House.

Tuckman, S. (1981). *Interpersonal Communication*, 2e (eds. S.L. Tubbs and S. Moss). New York: Random House.

Turnbull, H.R. (2002). Impacts of poverty on quality of life in families of children with disabilities. *Exceptional Children* 68 (2): 151–170.

Unsworth, C.A. (2016). *Clinical Reasoning in Stroke Rehabilitation*, 4e. Edinburgh: Elsievier.

Uys, K. and Samuels, A. (2010). Early childhood intervention in South Africa minimising the impact of disabilities. In: *Occupational Therapy: An African Perspective* (eds. V.M. Alers and R.B. Crouch). Johannesburg: Sarah Shorten Publishers.

Van der Reyden, D. and Crouch, R. (2014). *Occupational Therapy in Psychiatry and Mental Health*, 5e. London: Wiley Blackwell.

Van der Reyden and Sherwood, W. (2019). Core constructs and concepts. In: *VdTMoCA. The vona du Toit Model of Creative Ability* (eds. D. Van der Reyden, D. Casteleijn, W. Sherwood and P. de Witt). Pretoria: Vona and Marie du Toit Foundation.

Van der Reyden, D., Casteleijn, D., Sherwood, W., and de Witt, P. (2019). *VdTMoCA. The vona du Toit Model of Creative Ability*. Pretoria: Vona and Marie du Toit Foundation.

Voce, A. and Ramukumba, A. (1997). Cultural considerations in occupational therapy. In: *Occupational Therapy in Psychiatry and Mental Health*, 3e (eds. R. Crouch and V. Alers). Johannesburg: Maskew Miller and Longman (Pty) Ltd.

WHO (2004). *World Report on Knowledge for a Better Health Summary.* Geneva: World Health Organisation.

Wilkinson, J. and Canter, S. (1982). *Social Skills Training Manual: Assessment, Programme Design and Management of Training.* Chichester: New York: John Wiley and Sons.

World Federation of Occupational Therapists (WFOT) (2002). Minimal standards for the education of occupational therapists. `http:// www.wfot.org?singleNews`.

Yalom, I.D. (1975). *The Theory and Practice of Group Psychotherapy.* New York: Basic Books.

Yalom, I.D. (1985). *The Theory and Practice of Group Psychotherapy*, 3e. New York: Basic Books.

Index